U.S. Department
of Transportation
**Federal Railroad
Administration**

Human Factors Phase III:
Effects of Train Control Technology on
Operator Performance

Office of Research
and Development
Washington, DC 20590

U.S. Department of Transportation
Research and Special Programs Administration
John A. Volpe National Transportation Systems Center
Cambridge, MA 02142

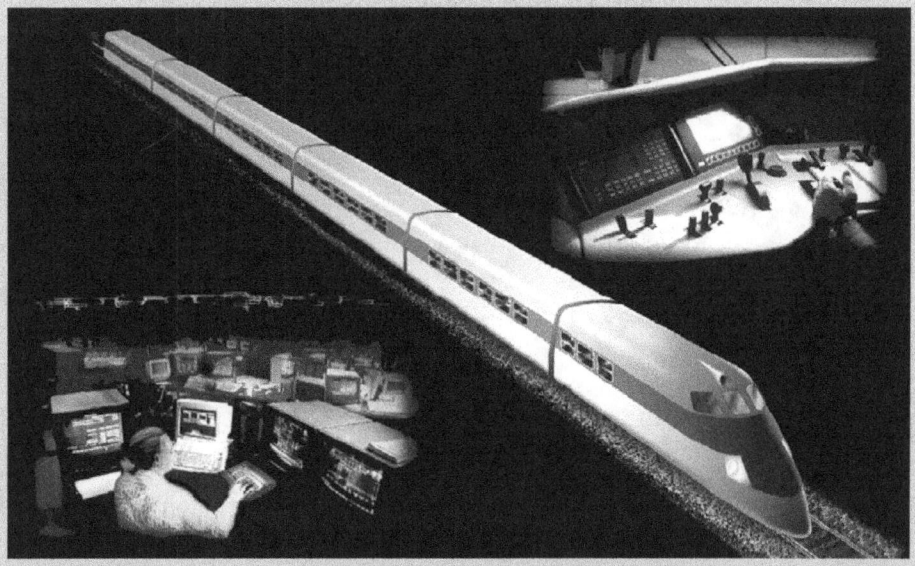

Human Factors in Railroad Operations

DOT/FRA/ORD-04/18

Final Report
January 2005

This document is available to the
public through the National Technical
Information Service, Springfield, VA 22161
This document is also available on
the FRA website at www.fra.dot.gov

REPORT DOCUMENTATION PAGE

Form Approved
OMB No. 0704-0188

1. AGENCY USE ONLY (*LEAVE BLANK*)	2. REPORT DATE January 2005	3. REPORT TYPE AND DATES COVERED Final Report August 1993 - July 1997

4. TITLE AND SUBTITLE Human Factors Phase III: Effects of Train Control Technology on Operator Performance	5. FUNDING NUMBERS R2103/RR204

6. AUTHOR(S)
Edward J. Lanzilotta and Thomas B. Sheridan

7. PERFORMING ORGANIZATION NAME(S) AND ADDRESS(ES) *Human-Machine Systems Laboratory Massachusetts Institute of Technology Cambridge, MA 02139	8. PERFORMING ORGANIZATION DOT-VNTSC-FRA-05-01

9. SPONSORING/MONITORING AGENCY NAME(S) AND ADDRESS(ES) U.S. Department of Transportation Federal Railroad Administration Office of Research and Development Mail Stop 20 1120 Vermont Avenue, NW Washington, DC 20590	10. SPONSORING/MONITORING AGENCY REPORT NUMBER DOT/FRA/ORD-04/18

11. SUPPLEMENTARY NOTES
Safety of High Speed Ground Transportation Systems Series

* Under Contract to: U.S. Department of Transportation
Research and Special Programs Administration
John A. Volpe National Transportation Systems Center
Cambridge, MA 02142-1093

12a. DISTRIBUTION/AVAILABILITY STATEMENT This document is available to the public through the National Technical Information Service, Springfield, VA 22161. This document is also available on the FRA web site at www.fra.dot.gov.	12b. DISTRIBUTION CODE

13. ABSTRACT (Maximum 200 words)

This report describes a study evaluating the effects of train control technology on locomotive engineer performance. Several types of train control systems were evaluated: partial automation (cruise control and programmed stop) and full automation were compared to manual train control. The study evaluated how these systems affected human performance related to position control, speed regulation and response to system failures, using a human-in-the-loop locomotive simulator.

The study found a significant difference in the variance of response times to brake failures and traction motor failures for the partial automation condition compared to manual and full automation conditions. In this condition, participants biased toward monitoring events outside the locomotive instead of the instrument panel.

14. SUBJECT TERMS automation, high-speed trains, human factors, human-in-the-loop simulation, risk estimation, safety, supervisory controls, train control, transportation	15. NUMBER OF PAGES 88
	16. PRICE CODE

17. SECURITY CLASSIFICATION OF REPORT Unclassified	18. SECURITY CLASSIFICATION OF THIS PAGE Unclassified	19. SECURITY CLASSIFICATION OF ABSTRACT Unclassified	LIMITATION OF ABSTRACT Unclassified

METRIC/ENGLISH CONVERSION FACTORS

ENGLISH TO METRIC

LENGTH (APPROXIMATE)

1 inch (in) = 2.5 centimeters (cm)
1 foot (ft) = 30 centimeters (cm)
1 yard (yd) = 0.9 meter (m)
1 mile (mi) = 1.6 kilometers (km)

AREA (APPROXIMATE)

1 square inch (sq in, in^2) = 6.5 square centimeters (cm^2)
1 square foot (sq ft, ft^2) = 0.09 square meter (m^2)
1 square yard (sq yd, yd^2) = 0.8 square meter (m^2)
1 square mile (sq mi, mi^2) = 2.6 square kilometers (km^2)
1 acre = 0.4 hectare (he) = 4,000 square meters (m^2)

MASS - WEIGHT (APPROXIMATE)

1 ounce (oz) = 28 grams (gm)
1 pound (lb) = 0.45 kilogram (kg)
1 short ton = 2,000 pounds (lb) = 0.9 tonne (t)

VOLUME (APPROXIMATE)

1 teaspoon (tsp) = 5 milliliters (ml)
1 tablespoon (tbsp) = 15 milliliters (ml)
1 fluid ounce (fl oz) = 30 milliliters (ml)
1 cup (c) = 0.24 liter (l)
1 pint (pt) = 0.47 liter (l)
1 quart (qt) = 0.96 liter (l)
1 gallon (gal) = 3.8 liters (l)
1 cubic foot (cu ft, ft^3) = 0.03 cubic meter (m^3)
1 cubic yard (cu yd, yd^3) = 0.76 cubic meter (m^3)

TEMPERATURE (EXACT)

$[(x-32)(5/9)]$ °F = y °C

METRIC TO ENGLISH

LENGTH (APPROXIMATE)

1 millimeter (mm) = 0.04 inch (in)
1 centimeter (cm) = 0.4 inch (in)
1 meter (m) = 3.3 feet (ft)
1 meter (m) = 1.1 yards (yd)
1 kilometer (km) = 0.6 mile (mi)

AREA (APPROXIMATE)

1 square centimeter (cm^2) = 0.16 square inch (sq in, in^2)
1 square meter (m^2) = 1.2 square yards (sq yd, yd^2)
1 square kilometer (km^2) = 0.4 square mile (sq mi, mi^2)
10,000 square meters (m^2) = 1 hectare (ha) = 2.5 acres

MASS - WEIGHT (APPROXIMATE)

1 gram (gm) = 0.036 ounce (oz)
1 kilogram (kg) = 2.2 pounds (lb)
1 tonne (t) = 1,000 kilograms (kg)
 = 1.1 short tons

VOLUME (APPROXIMATE)

1 milliliter (ml) = 0.03 fluid ounce (fl oz)
1 liter (l) = 2.1 pints (pt)
1 liter (l) = 1.06 quarts (qt)
1 liter (l) = 0.26 gallon (gal)
1 cubic meter (m^3) = 36 cubic feet (cu ft, ft^3)
1 cubic meter (m^3) = 1.3 cubic yards (cu yd, yd^3)

TEMPERATURE (EXACT)

$[(9/5) y + 32]$ °C = x °F

QUICK INCH - CENTIMETER LENGTH CONVERSION

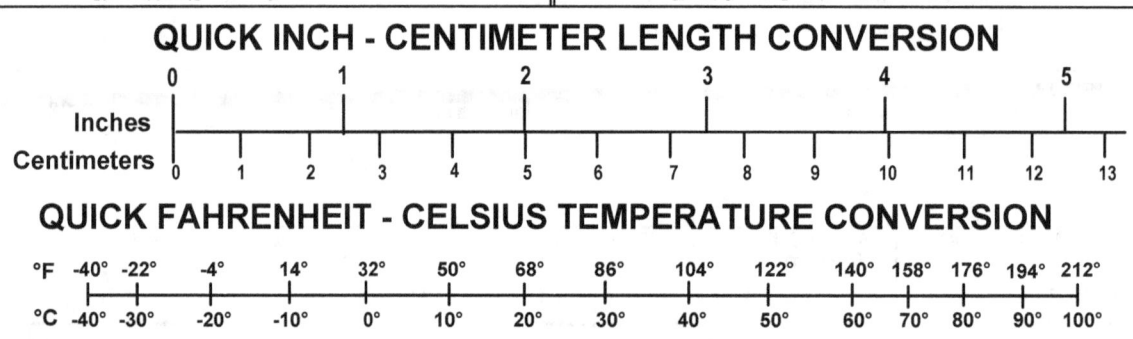

QUICK FAHRENHEIT - CELSIUS TEMPERATURE CONVERSION

°F	-40°	-22°	-4°	14°	32°	50°	68°	86°	104°	122°	140°	158°	176°	194°	212°
°C	-40°	-30°	-20°	-10°	0°	10°	20°	30°	40°	50°	60°	70°	80°	90°	100°

For more exact and or other conversion factors, see NIST Miscellaneous Publication 286, Units of Weights and Measures. Price $2.50
SD Catalog No. C13 10286

Updated 6/17/98

ii

PREFACE

This report summarizes work performed under an ongoing research program at the Volpe National Transportation Systems Center, Cambridge, Massachusetts, in collaboration with the Human-Machine Systems Laboratory at the Massachusetts Institute of Technology (Cambridge, Massachusetts). Supported by the Office of Research and Development, Federal Railroad Administration, the program is part of a comprehensive effort to identify and develop the technical information required for safety regulation of high-speed ground transportation. This is a final report on one component of the overall research program.

As vehicle speed increases, the information processing demands on the locomotive engineer become more significant. Relevant information is presented to the sensory systems at a higher rate, thereby reducing the available latency time for decisions and control actuation. To ensure that the engineer can adequately control the vehicle, human factors issues relative to this task must be sufficiently investigated. An earlier component of this research identified the task requirements of the locomotive engineers and central traffic control operators (Sheridan et al., 1994). This work also included review of the operator tasks in existing high-speed rail systems throughout the world.

More recent efforts focused on locomotive engineer performance and determined that there are two categories of operator aids most likely to be implemented in actual vehicles: advanced display-based decision aids, and advanced supervisory control. In the first case, the engineer is provided with additional information via advanced display technology, with the intent of improving the planning and decision capabilities of the engineer while underway. The second approach provides the engineer with supervisory control systems that reduce the required decision and actuation task load.

Simulation experiments have been conducted to explore the effects of these aids on operator performance. In order to determine the individual effects of each type of aid, separate experiments were conducted for each. The results of the experiment that evaluated the decision aids were reported in (Askey and Sheridan, 1996). This report focuses on the human factors issues of advanced supervisory control. In particular, this work addresses the effects of supervisory control on operator performance.

A companion report describes the theoretical development and experimental demonstration of the safety state model (Lanzilotta, 1996). The safety state model is a stochastic model of human-machine system behavior. The model utilizes a finite discrete Markov process to estimate the dynamic risk probability as a function of system state. The model is calibrated using observational data from an operational system. Application of the model is demonstrated through application to high-speed rail systems, using data obtained in the experiment described in this report.

Thus, the supervisory control experiment serves a dual purpose. First, it is a human behavioral study in the effects of supervisory control on human operator behavior in high-speed rail systems. Second, the experiment is a data generator for demonstration of a novel technique for estimating dynamic risk probability.

ACKNOWLEDGMENTS

The authors would like to acknowledge and thank the many people who were involved with and contributed to the completion of this work. In particular, we would like to thank Dr. Thomas Raslear of the Federal Railroad Administration for his guidance and support. Dr. Donald Sussman and Mr. Robert Dorer, at the Volpe National Transportation Systems Center (Volpe Center), lent significant contributions to the shape and direction of the work, and were able to provide key contacts and references. In addition, we would like to thank Dr. Peter Mengert and Mr. Robert DiSario for graciously sharing their knowledge and experience in matters of statistical analysis and experiment design. Mr. J. K. Pollard was instrumental in building the simulator throttle.

At the Massachusetts Institute of Technology, we would like to thank our colleagues in the Human-Machine Systems Laboratory for their contributions and support. Through collaborative work in simulation system development and complementary experimental work, my association with Ms. Shumei Yin Askey was fruitful and enlightening. Mr. Nicholas Patrick was especially helpful with statistical analysis and interpretation. Messrs. Jacob Einhorn, Bernardo Aumond, Steven Villareal, and Helias Marinakos have all been of assistance while in the process of taking on the next phases of the project. Our undergraduate assistants, Ms. Sapna Augustine, Ms. Wendy Chang, Ms. Grace Park, Mr. Joseph Wenish, and Ms. Jill Chen, were helpful in preparing for and conducting the experimental portion of the research. Dr. Jie Ren built the analog-to-digital converter used with the simulator throttle.

We would also like to acknowledge Messrs. John Tolman, George Newman, and Walter Nutter, of the Brotherhood of Locomotive Engineers, for their input during focus group discussions. Mr. Dennis Coffey and the Massachusetts Department of Transportation and Mr. Jack Flaherty of the Massachusetts Bay Transportation Authority were instrumental in arranging head-end rides, which provided valuable hands-on experience for the authors. Mr. Stephen Jones organized a visit to the Amtrak Centralized Traffic and Electrification Control facility.

Finally, special thanks to Dr. Judith Bürki-Cohen, of the Volpe Center, for her guidance and enthusiasm throughout this work. Her experience in experimental research was invaluable throughout the project, and was, along with her editorial input, critical to the successful completion of the experiments and subsequent reports.

TABLE OF CONTENTS

LIST OF FIGURES

LIST OF TABLES

EXECUTIVE SUMMARY

This report describes the motivation, background, and results of a set of experiments that evaluated the effects of supervisory control on the performance of locomotive engineers in high-speed train operations.

Control automation specifically refers to automatic devices designed to perform the fundamental tasks of vehicle control. These tasks include speed regulation (between stations) and position control (within stations). Three types of automatic control systems were considered: cruise control, programmed stop, and autopilot. A cruise control system maintains a constant speed, which is set by the engineer. A programmed stop system stops the vehicle at a precise location within the station—the engineer merely invokes the system under a set of prescribed circumstances to achieve accurate stopping performance. An autopilot system regulates the vehicle speed such that it follows a pre-programmed speed trajectory (as a function of vehicle position), and meets a set of pre-programmed stopping points. Once the vehicle is in motion and under autopilot control, no further input is required for standard operation.

As the level of supervisory control increases, the effect automation has on human operator performance when called upon to respond to emergency situations is unknown. Under fully manual operation, the engineer is responsible for speed regulation, position control, and system monitoring. In general rail vehicle operation, these tasks do not seem to present notably high mental workload levels. Increasing the level of supervisory control further lessens the engineer's workload. The result could lead to locomotive engineer performance improvement relative to system monitoring, due to greater availability of mental resources. On the other hand, the reduction in workload could result in a higher level of complacency or boredom, ultimately leading to a decrease in performance of the locomotive engineer relative to the system monitoring task.

Experimental work to explore this question was conducted using a laboratory-based simulation system. Twelve subjects drawn from the general student population were tested. Each subject had to undergo a 6-hour training course, to familiarize each of them with the locomotive engineers tasks. Each test subject then participated in a total of 9 hours of experimental tests, consisting of three individual 3-hour sessions. Each subject was given three variations of automation level: fully manual control, partial automation (cruise control and programmed stop), and full automation (autopilot). Each subject was exposed to the three treatments across three test sessions; each test session utilized only one treatment. The dependent variable was response to "unexpected" emergencies. Three emergencies were used: brake failure, traction motor failure, and grade crossing obstruction. All emergencies were recoverable (i.e., the test did not end upon the occurrence of an emergency). The responses to the emergencies were measured for both response time and response accuracy.

The results showed that there was a significant difference in the variance of response times to the brake failures and traction motor failures for the partial automation treatment when compared with the manual and full automation treatments. This suggests that, when using cruise control, the engineers had more of a tendency to bias their visual attention toward monitoring the external environment and away from the instrument panel. There was no significant difference found between the treatments (for either the mean response time or the response time variance) in the case of grade crossing obstruction. There was no significant difference in the response accuracy in any of the test comparisons.

The experimental results suggest that the use of cruise control reduces attention relative to failure detection indicated on the instrument panel. However, the experimental results also revealed that none of the treatments had an adverse effect on attention with respect to grade crossing obstructions. This finding is significant because, in general, grade crossings represent a significant risk in rail operations. No conclusions could be drawn with regard to response accuracy. The number of data points available from this experiment was not large enough to provide a statistically significant sample of data for such a comparison. In reviewing responses to a subjective rating questionnaire, it was concluded that the engineers believed full automation resulted in the lowest level of awareness, while the manual control treatment provided the highest level of awareness.

1. INTRODUCTION

As the United States moves toward high-speed passenger rail service, questions emerge regarding the usefulness and implications of vehicle automation. Study of existing foreign high-speed passenger rail operations, Train à Grande Vitesse (TGV) in France, Inter-City Express (ICE) in Germany, and Shinkansen in Japan, shows that implementing automation in these systems differ in degree and philosophy. In particular, the ICE embraces a high degree of automation; the TGV system provides the engineer with more advanced electronic assistance while retaining a high human interaction level for vehicle control (Bing, 1990).

Incorporating automation in rail vehicles simplifies the task of train operation while gaining greater consistency in overall system performance. The primary task in rail vehicle operation is speed control. Automating the speed control task will allow the engineer to focus on higher-level tasks, including monitoring for vehicle failures and other emergencies. The implication is increased use of automation will improve the overall performance of the locomotive engineer and the system.

The goal of this research is to gain a better understanding of the implications of supervisory control on human operator performance. Any automatic system will necessarily be designed to a set of performance criteria, and a successful implementation will meet those criteria. However, in introducing automation into the human machine system, the automatic systems change the nature of the interaction between the human and the machine. While in manual control, the engineer interacts directly with the vehicle; with supervisory control, the task of the locomotive engineer becomes a monitoring task, leading to a more indirect role of the engineer in vehicle control. Automation has potential implications in the areas of system safety and overall system performance; in addition, there are issues relative to task loading, complacency, and training of locomotive engineers.

Concerns identified include the effects of differing levels of supervisory control on human operator monitoring and intervention performance, as well as related effects on overall system performance. If introducing automation results in perfect "operator performance" as it is traditionally measured (for example, station-stopping performance or schedule maintenance) but degrades the overall system performance (for example, with regard to safety), this is a negative overall system impact.

System performance with respect to safety is of particular concern. Logically, perfect operator performance should result in perfect system performance with regard to safety, provided the operator performance is appropriately defined and measured. However, vehicle automation systems are designed to improve the traditional measures of operator performance, such as station stopping and schedule keeping. In the absence of an appropriate measure of operator performance relative to safety, it is possible that an automation system could improve the operator performance according to the traditional measures while adversely affecting overall system safety.

Early in this work, vehicle automation was divided into two broad categories. If you imagine the locomotive engineer as a component of a closed-loop control system (Figure 1), you will observe a *perception-decision-actuation* paradigm—the engineer perceives the state of the vehicle and environment, decides on a course of action, and takes action through the available vehicle controls (actuators). Typically, the engineer learned the operating rules through formal training. The perceived state of the vehicle and environment is compared to the allowed states governed by the operating rules, and any perceived differences are cause for a decision process, culminating in a plan of action modifying the vehicle state.

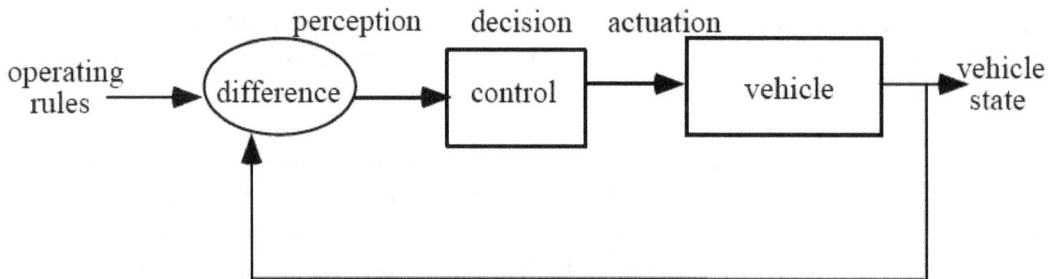

Figure 1. Closed-Loop Vehicle Control

Two of the most significant subtasks performed by the engineer are data gathering (perception) and control command (decision). Data gathering is the process of observing and interpreting available vehicle and system state information. State information may be obtained from in-vehicle instruments or displays, or it may be observed on wayside signals or signs. The data gathering generally occurs through the visual and aural information channels. Control command is the process of using the observed and interpreted data in conjunction with the operating rules and regulations, to make a control decision and perform the actuation required to implement that control decision. The control command process generally involves physical interaction between the engineer and the vehicle, typically through throttle and brake levers and control buttons.

Data gathering and control command together form the basis of operator-based closed-loop speed and position control. Speed control involves regulating the vehicle speed such that the vehicle complies with schedule and speed limit constraints. These two constraints run counter to one other. Tighter schedules imply higher speeds, while speed limits restrict the vehicle speed in the interest of safety. An optimum schedule minimizes the travel time without requiring speed in excess of known fixed speed limits. Position control involves stopping the vehicle at prescribed stop points, typically at stations or terminals. The significance of data gathering and control command subtasks is supported by a task analysis of the locomotive engineer, as performed in the early part of this research (Sheridan et al., 1994).

Based on this task division, automation in the cab can be separated into display automation and supervisory control. Display automation modifies the data gathering process, while supervisory control modifies the control command process. With increased levels of display automation, the information presented to the locomotive engineer includes higher levels of processing that otherwise might be performed internally by the engineer. For example, adding a preview display provides advance information about the track ahead, even if this portion of the track is out of visible range. A predictor display provides advance information on the vehicle state trajectory, based on the current vehicle and control states. An advisor display provides a suggested vehicle state trajectory, optimized for various constraints. The combination of these three systems provides the locomotive engineer with a powerful set of tools for improving performance.

The human performance concern, with regard to display automation, is potential overload of the operator sensory channels. Too much information will ultimately degrade overall performance due to the inability to process that information and extract the pertinent data from it. Experimental research in this area is part of the overall research project task reported in Askey and Sheridan (1996) and Askey (1995).

With supervisory control, an automatic system assumes the control of vehicle speed and position. The three types of supervisory control expected in high-speed rail systems are cruise control, programmed stop, and autopilot. A cruise control system is designed to maintain a constant speed set by the locomotive engineer, functionality similar to automobile cruise control systems. This frees the engineer from regulating vehicle speed in normal operational scenarios. However, the engineer still must monitor the wayside (for observation of speed limit indicators, such as signals and block markers) and vehicle systems (for observation of cruise control status, such as set speed), and the engineer must be ready to take control of the vehicle if the situation warrants. A programmed stop system will stop the vehicle at a pre-specified position, typically at a station. An autopilot is similar to cruise control, except that the desired speed is pre-programmed as a function of vehicle position. In addition, an autopilot incorporates the programmed stop for automatic station stopping.

The human performance concern, with respect to supervisory control, is that the engineer's situation awareness may be reduced as automation systems assume more of the control task. This reduction in situation awareness, characterized as an "out-of-the-loop" situation, is where the engineer is no longer actively involved with the immediate task. The implication is that in the event of an emergency or fault situation, the operator may consume precious response time trying to gain a perspective on the system state that might require the engineer to take control of the vehicle from the automation system, resulting in a delayed response. In addition, the engineer may respond in an inappropriate manner as a result of being "out-of-the-loop." Thus, the "operator out-of-the-loop" situation poses serious safety implications.

The goal of this work is to investigate the relationship between supervisory control and performance of the locomotive engineer in high-speed rail vehicles. Of particular interest are the effects of supervisory control on operator attentiveness and situation awareness. Much situation awareness work comes from the perspective of aircraft control. Characteristics of aircraft include rapid motion, highly dynamic scenario evolution, and the potential for grave consequences in the event of an accident, characteristics especially suitable for the study of situation awareness. With increasing levels of supervisory control and display aids in aircraft cockpits, there is heightened concern that the operator will lose perspective and awareness of the vehicle and environment states, and thus compromise the ability to operate the vehicle.

As rail vehicles move into high-speed operation, with speeds approaching or exceeding 186 mph (300 km/h), the concerns become similar to those of aircraft. High speed and momentum carry the risk of grave consequences in the event of a collision. In addition, the related high rate of ground coverage, along with increasing levels of automation and other forms of operator aids, increase the risk of operator error and resultant accident. This is of concern especially when automation transforms the task of the locomotive engineer from actuator control to instrument monitoring, thus lowering the level of direct interaction.

In the human factors research literature, the concept, definition, and measurement of situation awareness remains a topic of debate (Endsley, 1987; Endsley, 1988; Endsley, 1995; Gaba, et al., 1995; Hendy, 1995; Smith and Hancock, 1995; Sarter and Woods, 1995). For the purpose of this research, situation awareness was considered to be a useful qualitative concept for discussing the effects of automation. The overall notion that situation awareness includes the adaptive coupling between humans and machines is of central importance. However, many of the techniques currently available for evaluating situation awareness incur some level of intrusiveness into the operational scenario. The experiment described herein uses emergency response measurement in an effort to avoid the problem of task intrusion.

Attention allocation is a research area related to situation awareness. Operator attention is a limited resource which is dynamically allocated. There are three categories of attention allocation: selective attention, focused attention, and divided attention (Sanders and McCormick, 1987; Wickens, 1992). With *selective attention*, an operator monitors several sources of information, looking for the occurrence of particular events. The *load stress* increases with an increasing number of channels of information, while the *speed stress* increases by increasing the information rate. According to work by Goldstein and Dorfman (1978), load stress is more likely to degrade performance than speed stress. *Focused attention* occurs when an operator attempts to monitor a few information sources, often in the presence of distracting noise. The noise is considered information on other channels—focused attention is the process of "tuning out" the less important information in favor of the more critical information. If competing information occurs in the visual mode, spatial proximity of the two sources of information can degrade focused attention. *Divided attention*, also termed *timesharing*, occurs when an operator must perform more than one task at a given time. Divided attention differs from selective attention in that the operator is actively performing useful work while monitoring information sources; with selective attention, the primary task is information monitoring. There is general agreement that there is limited human capacity for divided attention, although cognitive psychologists have a variety of theories for describing the mechanisms involved (Senders, 1964; Wickens, 1994; Sanders and McCormick, 1987). Despite the theories and classifications of attention allocation, much remains unknown. Sanders and McCormick (1987) succinctly state: "Even with all the theory building and research in the area of divided attention, there is still much we do not understand. How these factors come together to influence performance is still not entirely clear. Predictions on the outcome of timesharing real-world tasks, therefore, are still relatively primitive."

Regardless of the theoretical models, a practical issue relative to operation of high-speed rail vehicles remains: How does the transition to higher speeds affect the ability of a locomotive engineer to obtain, interpret, and act on information pertinent to vehicle operation? When engineers monitor one or more displays, they should view (sample) each display frequently enough and for sufficient duration to extract the information presented. Typically, the monitoring field of the engineer is distributed across two broad areas of potential visual focus: the instrument panel (located within the cab, also known as the dashboard), and the environment outside the cab. The focal distances of the two focus areas differ enough that it is generally difficult for an engineer to have concurrent visual focus on both. As a result, the engineer must alternate his visual attention between the instrument panel and the external environment. The instruments on the dashboard are considered to be displays in the typical human factors sense;

we can also consider the external view to be a "display," as it could be implemented with a camera and monitor screen in place of a traditional window.

Operating a rail vehicle (and, in general, operating any vehicle) can be considered a combination of divided attention and selective attention tasks. The task is divided attention, in that the locomotive engineer must attend to several different tasks at once, including speed control, position control, system status monitoring, and vehicle status monitoring. The monitoring subtasks can each be considered as selective attention tasks. The objective is to identify a system or vehicle fault, and the engineer must monitor several channels of information to detect a fault. From a different perspective, the task of a locomotive engineer is a combination of relatively high frequency monitoring and control (to fulfill the task of speed and position control) with vigilance (for system failures and emergencies).

Attention bias is the degree to which the operator's attention is allocated within an attention classification scheme. For rail vehicle operation, allocation of attention is discussed in several areas: separate visual focus areas (in-cab instrument versus external environment), separate types of attention allocation (divided attention versus selective attention), and different levels of information bandwidth (monitoring versus vigilance).

Introducing supervisory control at high speed has the potential for significantly altering the role of the locomotive engineer. Potential effects include degrading situation awareness and attention allocation, as well as increasing fatigue, complacency, and boredom. The experimental work described in this report determined the extent of the impact on human performance by incorporating supervisory control in high-speed rail. Subjects were asked to operate a passenger train in a high-speed rail simulation system, according to a set of operating rules and schedule. The subjects performed three separate test runs, each with a different level of supervisory control. During the test runs, the subjects were exposed to various emergency situations requiring active response. Response times and response accuracy to these emergencies were measured and compared. The hypothesis is that increasing the level of supervisory control will have a significant effect on the attention bias of the engineer, and the overall effect of supervisory control on engineer response will depend on the significance level of the emergency.

2. METHOD

2.1 High-Speed Rail Simulation System

The High-Speed Rail Simulation System was used to conduct the experiment. This system is a human-in-the-loop simulator designed for use in human factors experiments. Through a modular design philosophy, this system can be reconfigured for a variety of experimental needs. The following sections describe the configuration used for the supervisory control experiment. For a more detailed description of the design and implementation of the high-speed rail simulation, see Appendix A of Lanzilotta, 1996.

2.1.1 System Configuration

The simulation system operated on a set of Silicon Graphics graphics workstations, which communicated via a local area network. The system used C programming language and ran under the Irix operating system. For the experiment described in this report, the system configuration utilized three workstations (Figure 2) manufactured by Silicon Graphics, Inc. (SGI). The workstations included one Indigo-2 model and two Personal Iris machines.

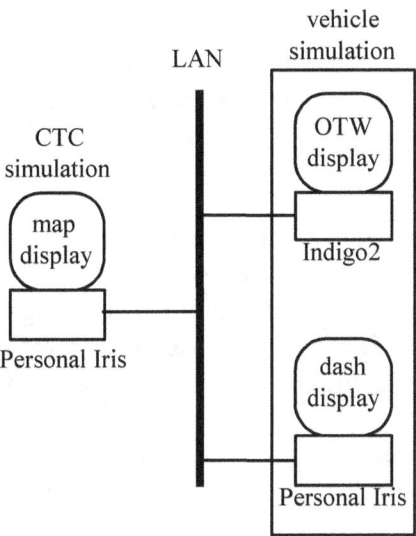

Figure 2. Simulation System Configuration

One Personal Iris was configured as the Central Traffic Control (CTC) operator interface. The experimenter operated this machine. The CTC operator (also called the dispatcher) normally monitors the overall state of the system, controlling the state of the switches, and acts as supervisor for the vehicles in the system. The primary display at this interface was a plan-view map of the rail system. Figure 2 depicts this workstation on the left, and describes its function (CTC) and display features.

The train simulation required the use of two workstations. One workstation, an Indigo-2 (with Extreme graphics), provided the out-the-window (OTW) display. The software used to create the OTW view operated in conjunction with the vehicle dynamics computations. The other workstation, a Personal Iris, was configured as the instrument panel (dashboard) display. The

7

subjects acted as locomotive engineers, applying input via a control lever (used for the combined functionality of thrust and brake commands) and keyboard inputs. Figure 2 shows these two workstations on the right. The rectangular box around the two workstation icons shows that they have related functionality (vehicle simulation), while the individual icons identify the type of machine and display functions of each workstation.

The train cab environment in the simulation system consisted of two workstations on a large computer table. Mounted on the right-hand side of the table was a full-size throttle lever (adapted from a conventional boat throttle). The table was in an isolated room; partitions enclosed the test subject. The CTC operator environment consisted of a computer table and a single workstation.

2.1.2 Subject Interface

In addition to the two computer displays, computer keyboard, and control lever on the computer table, additional information was available to the test subjects on paper. This information could be used at their discretion, and included a map of the rail system, a summary of the operating schedule, and a summary of the rail signal codes.

The display on the left had a dedicated OTW view. The OTW view as designed is a night view of the environment, with objects lighted by the vehicle (e.g., a headlight). The rails and roadbed were drawn as fading into the distance. The roadbed included simple rock-like objects to provide a sense of motion, especially at lower vehicle speeds. In addition, the view of the rails was designed to vibrate with vehicle motion, with increasing amplitude at higher speeds, heightening the perception of speed.

Static objects in the environment appeared as wire-frame images. There were several types and sizes of objects, and simple object shapes combined to create more complex structures. Mileposts appeared as reflective black-on-white signs on the right side of the road, and block signals appeared overhead, with "light-emitting" signals and reflective identification numerals above. Grade crossings appeared as gray roadways, and the highway vehicles appeared as solid blue cars. Stations appeared as wire frame shapes, with purple and blue walls. When the front edge of the vehicle was within the boundaries of the station, a head-up display appeared on the windscreen, for the engineer to use as an aid for vehicle positioning in the station.[1]

The display on the right showed the vehicle's instrument panel, containing the gauges, displays, and warning lights available to the engineer (Figure A-3 on page 39). In the center of this display was a large round speedometer dial gauge. This gauge was calibrated to 217.5 mph (350 km/h), and had a red pointer to indicate current speed. A yellow pointer, located beneath the red pointer, indicated the controlled speed when the vehicle was operating in one of the automation modes (cruise control, programmed stop, or autopilot). Four smaller round gauges displayed system values, including brake tank pressure (two gauges), wheel bearing temperature, and power supply voltage. Three color-coded indicator lights showed automation mode engagement. Four vertical LED-bar indicators indicated the current level applied to the four traction motors. Four

---

[1] Locomotive engineers normally look out the side window to obtain information to brake as a station is approached. The part-task simulator had no window to see the boundaries of the station, so the information they were missing was given in the head-up display.

color-coded indicator lights showed other vehicle warnings and status, including ATP system warning/penalty, emergency brake activation, alerter system warning/penalty, and door status. In-cab signaling provided for both the currently occupied block and the next approaching block. A text display was used for the communication channel. A digital system clock was provided.

The primary input device was a combination control lever. Built from a modified boat throttle and mounted into the computer table, the subject used this control to issue thrust and brake commands to the vehicle. The full forward position (i.e., away from the engineer), applied maximum thrust to the vehicle. Conversely, in the full backward position, maximum braking was applied. A detent in the center of travel was used for coasting. The control lever was connected to a potentiometer, which controlled a voltage converted by an analog-to-digital (A/D) converter into a digital number. The digital form of the control command was sent, via a serial link, to the workstation for use in the vehicle dynamics software.

All other engineer input was performed through the computer keyboard. The top row of function keys acted as control buttons for a variety of vehicle functions, including alerter response, automation mode enable, motor circuit breaker reset, brake system reset, door control, manual control of emergency braking, and emergency brake reset. The "arrow" keys ("up-arrow" and "down-arrow") controlled the set speed in cruise control mode. In addition, the alphanumeric keys were used to type messages in the communications channel.

2.1.3 Design and Implementation of Control Automation Systems

Included in the train simulation were three supervisory control systems: cruise control, programmed stop, and autopilot.

The cruise-control system was designed to maintain a constant, operator-selected speed. The system was engaged by depressing the appropriate control button, which maintained the current vehicle speed. The set speed was modulated via the up-down arrow keys on the keyboard. The controller was implemented as a proportional-integral (PI) controller that regulates speed, using thrust only. Manual application of service brakes disengaged the cruise control system.

The programmed stop system was designed to stop the vehicle at the end of the current block. It was, in effect, a closed-loop position control system. Depressing the appropriate control button engaged the system. If engaged properly, the system stopped the vehicle using a brake curve lookup table to determine braking force. Several safeguards protected against improper usage: 1) the engagement speed must be below 49.7 mph (80 km/h), and 2) the distance to the stop point must exceed the minimum required braking distance. Violating either of these conditions caused the emergency brakes to be applied. During normal operation of the programmed stop system, manually applying the service brakes disengaged the programmed stop system.

The autopilot was a speed regulation system, similar to the cruise-control system. Depressing the appropriate control button engaged the system. The set speed was pre-programmed as a speed trajectory function of vehicle position. The controller was implemented as a PI controller for thrust and brakes, in conjunction with the programmed stop system in the vicinity of stations. Manually applying the service brakes disengaged the autopilot system.

2.2 Experiment Design

2.2.1 Subject Task

At the highest level, the task was to control a simulated rail vehicle through a virtual rail system. The objective was to involve the subject to the highest degree possible, in the task of a locomotive engineer. This overall task has two components—vehicle control and system monitoring. Vehicle control includes active participation on the part of the human, by manipulating control levers and switches; system monitoring is entirely passive.

Vehicle control consists of speed and position control of the vehicle. Vehicle speed is regulated through monitoring of speed and active response using the throttle and brake, to meet conflicting constraints of schedule requirements and speed limits. Position control occurs when stopping the vehicle at stations and terminals. The level of vehicle control varied for the subject as the level of supervisory control was varied in the experiment.

System monitoring included monitoring the vehicle systems. With respect to the vehicle systems, the subject monitored for brake and motor failures specifically, and system anomalies in general. The subject monitored the environment in which the train was passing, including observing passing mileposts (for position identification), block signals (for both position identification and signal observance), wayside landmarks (to identify braking points), and grade crossing status (to identify obstructions in the crossings). In addition, the subject monitored the vehicle speed and the in-cab signals at all times to determine whether current vehicle speed complied with applicable speed limits, regardless of the level of supervisory control in use.

The rail system used was a two-station shuttle system, separated by 31.1 mi (50 km) of track. Outside each station a looping section of track (with a switch) reversed the vehicle on the main track (see Figure A-1 on page 36). The one-way travel time between the two stations was approximately 18 minutes, and the travel time around the loop approximately 7 minutes. In each test session, the subject operated the vehicle on three roundtrip circuits of the system. Each test session required approximately 3 hours.

The subject controlled the speed (and consequently, the position) of the vehicle by applying either thrust or braking forces, through the combined control lever. The selected speed was subject to speed limit constraints that were due to either civil speed limits (static) or signal speed limits (dynamic). The selected speed was also subject to the prescribed schedule, implying that a minimum average speed be maintained over each trip leg.

2.2.2 Independent Variable

The independent variable for this experiment was the level of supervisory control. Three levels of automation were used: no automation (manual control only), partial automation (use of both cruise control and programmed stop), and full automation (autopilot).

Under manual control, the subject was required to perform all vehicle operation tasks, including monitoring vehicle speed, vehicle position, block signal states, determining block speed limits, and actuation of throttle and brake controls to vary vehicle speed. When using cruise control and programmed stop, the requirement for modulating the throttle and brake controls was removed, implicitly relaxing the requirement for monitoring the instantaneous vehicle speed. However, monitoring vehicle position, monitoring signal states, and selection of a desired speed were required tasks. In the case of autopilot operation, all normal speed regulation tasks were removed from the responsibility of the locomotive engineer, who was required to monitor only for and respond to emergency situations.

2.2.3 Dependent Variables

The primary dependent measure was response to unexpected failures. Two types of response measures were made at each failure point. One was the response time, which was measured from the onset of the failure to the proper action taken in response to that failure. The response time could vary as a result of perception, decision, or action latencies, or any combination of the three. The second measure was a rating of the accuracy or correctness of the response. This measure is, by nature, more qualitative than the response time measure.

2.2.4 Subject Counterbalancing

To counterbalance possible learning effects, the presentation order of the automation level was counterbalanced among each group of six subjects. That is, each subject within a group of six experienced the three automation modes in a different order. The resultant design appears in Table 1.

Table 1 identifies the counterbalancing design for a within-subject, three-treatment experiment. Such an experiment has six different variants of treatment presentation order. As a result, six subjects formed a counterbalance group. Each subject test session is known as a *shift*, and the *shift number* represents the relative shift count for each individual subject. For example, Subject 1 was asked to use manual mode for the entire first shift, partial automation for Shift 2, followed by full automation in Shift 3.

The fourth column of Table 1 presents the failure scenarios. Each failure scenario represents a set of failures that occurred in a prescribed order at prescribed positions along the route. The failure scenarios were designed such that occurrence of failure events would be perceived to be random. The occurrences of failure types in the set of scenarios were distributed to reinforce the perception of randomness. The failure scenarios were not counterbalanced with respect to shift position. As a result, the failure scenarios are counterbalanced with respect to automation type. Two different sets of failure scenarios were utilized, dividing the 12 subjects into 2 groups of 6.

2.2.5 Failure Scenarios

Three different types of failure modes were possible during the test sessions: brake failure, motor failure, and grade crossing obstruction. Each represented a different type of detection-response paradigm. Two of the failure modes can be considered system failures, while the third is considered an environment failure.

The brake failure was the simplest type of failure. One of the brake reservoirs lost pressure, which was detected by a slowly dropping pressure on the brake reservoir pressure gauge. Switching to an alternate compressor (via a manually controlled switch on the control panel) rectified the fault. This failure had the simplest detection-response pattern—the detection was direct, via instrument panel gauges, and the response required one step. This is a vehicle system failure.

A motor failure was the other vehicle-based failure. In this scenario, the circuit breaker "tripped" for one motor (i.e., the circuit was broken, interrupting power to the motor). The circuit breaker had to be reset to restore motor operation. The failure was detected by a zero current reading on one of the motor ammeters located on the instrument panel. The response consisted of two steps: power to the motors had to be removed, and the appropriate circuit breaker reset switch had to be depressed. If the circuit breaker reset button was depressed before power was removed, all of the other circuit breakers would trip, necessitating reset of all the motors.

Table 1. Subject Counterbalancing

Subject Number	Shift Number	Automation Type	Failure Scenario
1	1	m	a
	2	p	b
	3	f	c
2	1	m	a
	2	f	b
	3	p	c
3	1	p	a
	2	m	b
	3	f	c
4	1	p	a
	2	f	b
	3	m	c
5	1	f	a
	2	m	b
	3	p	c
6	1	f	a
	2	p	b
	3	m	c

A grade crossing obstruction was the third failure. In this case, a car crossing the track became stuck while still partly in the crossing. The engineer had to identify that the car was stuck, and apply the brakes so that the train did not collide with the car. Depending on the speed of the train and the point at which the obstruction was detected the proper response could be either full service braking or emergency braking. Thus, this failure required a three-step detection-decision-action sequence: first, identifying the obstruction; then determining the proper braking strategy; then enacting the braking strategy. This failure was considered an environment failure.

The grade crossing failure also differed from the other two failures in that a strategy decision was required. The engineer determined the proximity of the danger, and chose a braking strategy based on an estimation of the danger status. In the other two failure scenarios, reacting to the failure was always the same; the engineer was only required to detect the failure and then correctly enact one possible course of action.

In the course of three test sessions, each subject experienced a total of six occurrences of each failure type. An important design goal was maintenance of the perception, from the perspective of the subjects, that the failures were generated randomly. This goal was subject to the constraint that the failures actually occur in fixed positions on the track, in order to maintain experimental control.

To meet these criteria, six track positions were designated for each failure type. The total number of failures in each test session would be four, six, or eight, as a function of the test number. Each counterbalanced group of six subjects (Section 2.2.4) received the same presentation of failures, with respect to relative test number. However, because of the counterbalancing design, the distribution of failure scenarios with respect to automation mode was also counterbalanced with respect to automation level. See Table 2 for the distribution of failure scenarios used in the experiment.

The notation used in the table is as follows: Each subject group consisted of a set of six subjects, with the order of automation counterbalanced as specified in Table 2. The individual failures are notated with the letter codes "o" for obstruction, "b" for brake failure, and "m" for motor failure. The numeral next to the letter code specifies the position on the track for the failure. For each round trip (consisting of two consecutive trip legs), six failure points were specified for each type of failure. Thus, the numeral corresponds to the relative position of the failure for that failure type. The failure points were specified such that the different failure types occurred at different points, precluding a combination failure.

Table 2. Failure Scenarios

Subject Group	Shift	Trip Leg 1,2	Trip Leg 3,4	Trip Leg 5,6
A	1	m2,b4	b3,m4,o4	o3,b5,m6
A	2	O5,b6	b2,o6	o2,m5
A	3	b1	m1	o1,m3
B	1	b2,o3	b4	m3
B	2	m1,o1,b6	m4,o4,b5	b1,m2
B	3	o2,b3	m6,o6	o5,m5

13

2.2.6 Performance Monitoring and Incentives

To ensure that proficiency of the test subject, relative to the tasks of a locomotive engineer, would not affect the test results (i.e., to assure that the test subjects were capable of adequately controlling the train), the performance of each test subject was monitored throughout the test sessions. A bonus system providing monetary rewards for good performance was a performance incentive for the subjects. In addition, penalties were assessed for prohibited behavior. At the end of each test session, the subject's performance was evaluated with regard to bonuses and penalties. A detailed discussion of the bonus and penalty points schedule is included in Appendix A. The bonus point schedules appear in Tables A-6 through A-8 on pages 58-60, and the penalty point schedules appear in Tables A-8 through A-10 on pages 60-61.

2.3 Subjects

In the course of the experiment, there were 12 paid subjects. An additional eight subjects were used for development of the training and test procedures. The subjects were selected from the MIT student population and no restrictions were placed on age or gender. The ages of the subject group ranged from (approximately) 19 to 35 years old. There were 16 undergraduate students, 3 graduate students, and 1 alumnus. The division by gender was 3 women and 17 men.

The basic criterion for subject selection was current or recent status as an MIT student. The proximity to an educational institution like MIT allowed access to a population that is enthusiastic about transportation and technology, reasonably well trained in the relevant principles of physics, and capable of rapid assimilation of technical material. No arbitrary limits were placed on academic experience. Instead, level of interest in the project was used as a filter, through the use of written preparatory material (described in Section 2.4.1).

2.4 Procedures

2.4.1 Training

To provide the subject candidates with sufficient background in rail systems operation, a written tutorial was prepared for their review. Tutorial material included general rail concepts (such as block signaling), implementation-specific design features (such as the available supervisory control modes), and experiment details (for example, training procedures and performance incentives). See Appendix A for the tutorial. Prior to scheduling an initial training session, tutorial material was distributed to subject candidates.

Written preparatory material served two purposes. One was the consistent and efficient presentation of fundamental concepts of rail operation. All potential subjects were exposed to the same material, in the same format. Second, the tutorial acted as a filter for subject interest in the project. Tutorial review required an investment on the part of the subject candidates. Those subject candidates not sufficiently interested were not inclined to continue with participation. As a result, the profile of the participating subjects was appropriately biased toward people interested in rail systems.

Subjects were trained to respond to failures through a variety of mechanisms. Details of the potential failures and the appropriate responses were included in the tutorial material. The subjects were then introduced to the failures by demonstration in the early part of the hands-on training procedures. Finally, near the end of the training procedures, subjects were given the opportunity to experience the failures and practice response to those failures.

Training for each subject was conducted over two sessions, each lasting 3 hours, on separate days. The first training session commenced with a brief written quiz, to gauge the subject's understanding of the tutorial. The quiz (Appendix B) consisted of 25 multiple-choice questions, and required approximately 10 minutes to complete. When completed, the experimenter and subject reviewed the quiz and discussed any problem areas. The first training session then continued with hands-on instruction on the simulator (Appendix E). The next half-hour period consisted of experimenter demonstrations of the displays and controls of the simulator, as well as the operational modes and automation systems. Strategies for operating the train and utilizing the automation were discussed. The subject was then instructed to take one solo, round-trip passage of the system. At this point, no failures were activated, and the experimenter acted as the CTC operator. Each subject subsequently performed a second solo, round-trip, with failures activated at expected points for practice.

The second training session was dedicated to practice and evaluation of manual control skills. Each subject was instructed to take a full three-round-trip shift using manual control only. The subjects were instructed to abide by the published schedule, and were informed that random failures might occur. The first hour was considered a practice period, during which the subjects were encouraged to experiment with strategies to improve their station stopping and schedule performance. The latter 2 hours of the shift were considered a road test, during which the performance of station stopping was measured. At the end of the shift, the station stopping performance was evaluated, and a recommendation for continuing with the test sessions was made, based on the results of this evaluation.

Criteria for subject continuation with the test portion were based on performance during the road test portion of the second training session. Acceptance criteria included station-stopping accuracy, with less than 32.8 ft (10 m) allowed for undershoot or overshoot as a requirement. In addition, the subjects were informed that any penalty applications of the emergency brake, due to the ATP or alerter systems, were not acceptable, and would result in disqualification. Schedule performance was measured during the road test and reviewed with the subjects after training was completed; however, schedule performance was not used as an objective criterion for evaluation during the road test sessions.

2.4.2 Tests

The test phase consisted of three separate test sessions termed *shifts* (described in Section 2.2.4). Each shift corresponded to an operating shift, during which the subject was expected to follow a 3-hour operating schedule. Only one level of automation was to be used throughout each shift. For example, if a subject was operating in a manual control shift, the use of any automation was prohibited for the duration of the shift.

2.4.3 Data Collection and Processing

In operating the vehicle simulator, a variety of vehicle state data were recorded. Each data record included a time stamp, an event code symbol, the total distance traveled, the current position (in terms of the current occupied block and the position within that block), and the current vehicle speed. With certain events, an optional field could be recorded. The disk file format used was ASCII text.

Data records indicating the vehicle position and speed were written continuously during the test runs, at the rate of one every 0.6 seconds. An additional field in this record, containing a number between 1.0 and -1.0, indicated the position of the combined control lever (and corresponding to maximum thrust and maximum brake, respectively). In the event that the engineer was moving the control lever, the write rate of these records was increased to capture all of the input of the test subject, to a maximum rate of the simulation cycle (60 milliseconds per cycle).

Data records also were written when the user depressed any of the control keys. These records, in conjunction with the vehicle state records, were used to identify the actions of the test subjects. Other data records were written whenever the vehicle changes operating state (e.g., when an automation mode was successfully engaged). Note that a distinction was made between an operator command that may result in vehicle state change, and the actual change of vehicle state resulting from the command. Separating the command from the state change allowed identification of erroneous operator input, as well as vehicle state changes that occurred independently of operator command.

After completing each subject test run, a raw data file was stored on disk. Each file contained all the events, as described in Section 3, recorded during the test run. The file format was ASCII text, and a typical data file for each 3-hour test run occupied approximately 1.5 MB. The data files were post-processed to extract the pertinent response data.

Immediately after the subject completed a test session, a program named BONUS processed the raw data file. This program calculated the bonus points that the subject earned throughout the test. In addition to the default mode, which identified station stop performance, schedule performance, and failure response performance, BONUS also included operating modes which allowed isolation of any of these categories of performance measurement. After the subjects were apprised of their BONUS performance, BONUS calculated and stored the stopping performance and schedule maintenance data in separate disk files.

A program named TRANSFORM calculated the response times and accuracy to the failure events. The output of this program is an ASCII data file containing the response time and accuracy for each failure experienced by the subject. Comparable data from the TRANSFORM output and the BONUS output were used for accuracy crosscheck and verification.

3. RESULTS

The experimental results were based on measuring subject response to unexpected emergencies during normal operation. Each subject session (*shift*) had a designated automation mode (manual, partial, or full), and the pattern of emergencies experienced during a shift depended on the *shift number* and *subject group*. As detailed in Section 2.2.4, the automation type was counterbalanced with respect to shift number. As a result, the failure patterns were counterbalanced with respect to automation type.

3.1 Response Time to Unexpected Failures

The primary measure used to compare subject performance was response time to unexpected failures using three distinct failure modes: brake failure, motor failure, and track obstruction. The response time was measured as the elapsed time between the onset of the failure and execution of the correct response to that failure. In the case of brake failure, brake pressure decreased at the onset of failure, and the correct response to depress the brake pump button on the dashboard. In the case of motor failure, the motor current was interrupted in one of the traction motors at the onset of failure, indicated by a zero current reading on the corresponding ammeter (on the instrument panel). The correct response was to restore motor power through reset of the appropriate motor circuit breaker. For track obstruction, the onset of the failure was defined as the moment the car stops on the track, and the correct response to apply either full service braking or the emergency brake.

Tables 3 through 5 illustrate an analysis of the measured response times for the 12 subjects. Due to the counterbalancing design, the exact number of failures of each type and under each treatment varied from subject to subject. The tables highlight the minimum and maximum response times for each failure, as well as the mean, standard deviation, and variance of each data set. Table 3 contains the response time data for the brake failures. Table 4 contains the response time data for the motor failures. Table 5 contains the response time data for the obstruction failures. Figures 3 through 5 display the data in box-plot representation (Tukey, 1977). The box-plot display includes a two-segment box, identifying the median value (represented by the center line) as well as the 25 and 75 percentile values (shown as the lower and upper edges of the box). The 25 and 75 percentile values also are known as *hinges*. The range between the hinges is the *H-spread*. The value of *one step* is calculated as 150 percent of the H-spread. The *inner fences* are defined as the bounds one step from the hinges. In the event that the data fell within the inner fences, the whiskers show the extent of the range. The crosses beyond the whiskers identify the *outliers*, which are data beyond the inner fences. In all the box-plot figures, automation level is labeled such that automation Level 1 corresponds to manual control, automation Level 2 refers to partial automation (cruise control and programmed stop), and automation Level 3 corresponds to full automation (autopilot).

Table 3. Response Time Data for Brake Failure

	Manual	Partial	Full
Min	5.5	5.6	4.4
Max	61.9	119.2	78.1
Mean	22.8	32.7	22.0
Standard Deviation	16.26	30.37	16.39
Variance	264.41	922.35	268.67

Table 4. Response Time Data for Motor Failure

	Manual	Partial	Full
Min	2.7	2.6	2.9
Max	78.7	122.6	38.6
Mean	11.4	20.1	12.7
Standard Deviation	15.11	29.49	10.62
Variance	228.28	869.67	112.75

Table 5. Response Time Data for Obstruction Failure

	Manual	Partial	Full
Min	0.9	1.0	1.3
Max	14.8	14.8	17.4
Mean	4.1	4.1	5.1
Standard Deviation	4.17	3.54	4.36
Variance	17.38	12.51	19.04

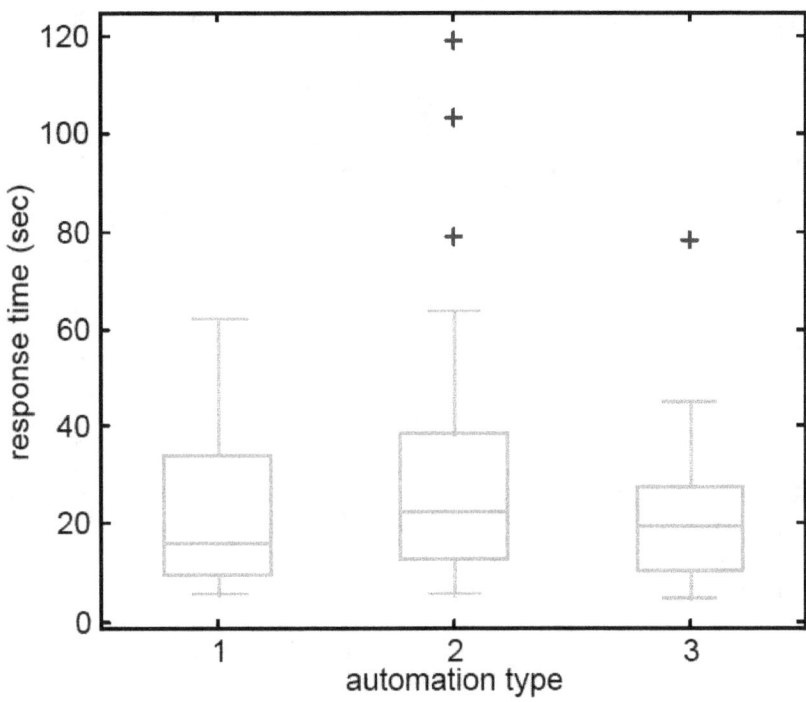

Figure 3. Box-Plot Display of Brake Failure Response Time

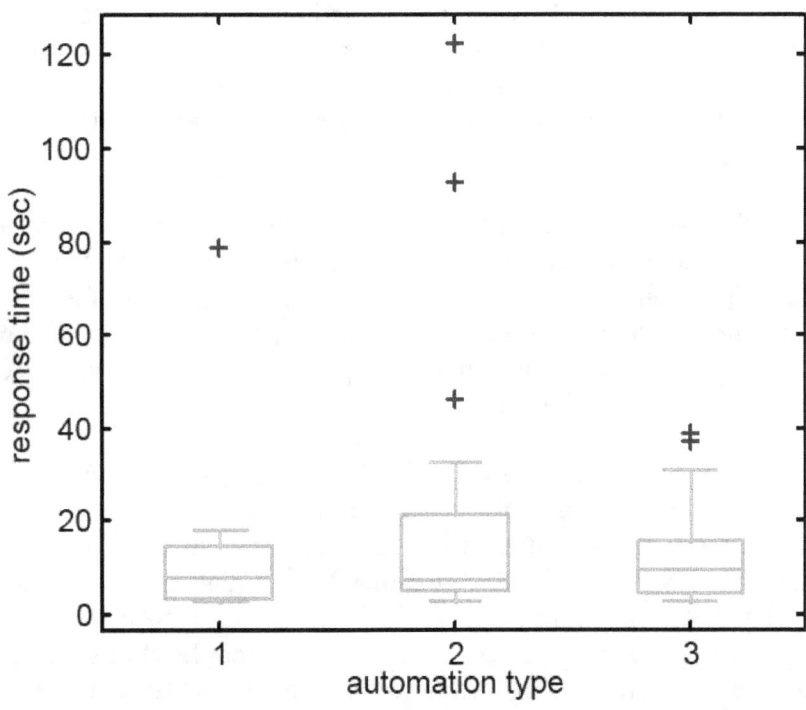

Figure 4. Box-Plot Display of Motor Failure Response Time

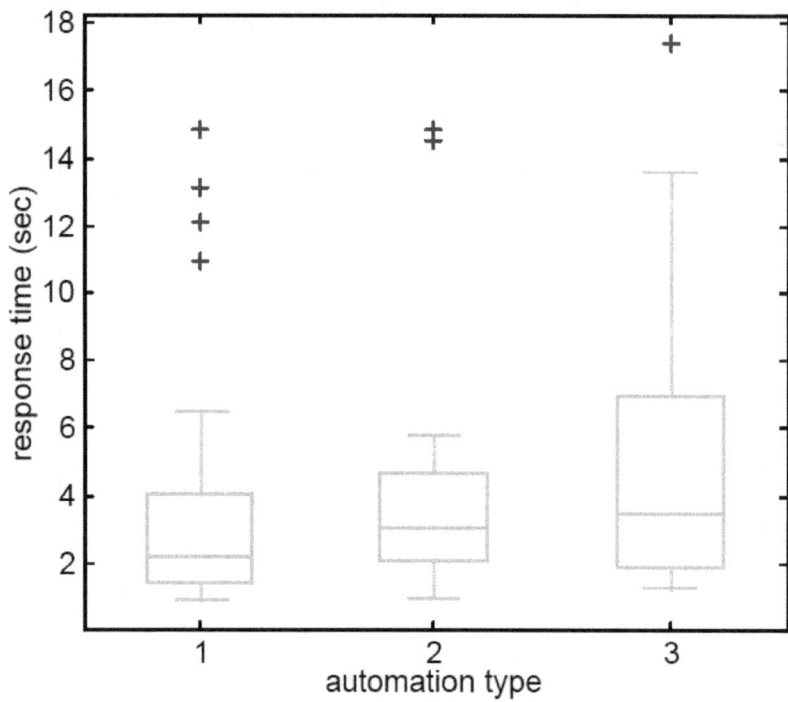

Figure 5. Box-Plot Display of Obstruction Failure Response Time

The scientific hypothesis postulates that there exists a difference in response time to unexpected failures, when comparing performance between the applied levels of supervisory control. The corresponding null hypothesis is that there are no differences in emergency response times, with respect to automation level. The related statistical null hypothesis is that there are no statistically significant differences in the response times; in other words, any observed differences are due to random sampling and measurement noise.

A typical approach would be to compare the mean response times, using a one-way analysis of variance (ANOVA) technique. However, the ANOVA technique assumes that the population variance of the different treatment populations is equal. A quick inspection of the sample variances (Tables 3 through 5) shows that observed variances are substantially different, leading to a suspicion that this data might not support the assumption. The observed variances are especially disparate in the cases of brake and motor failures.

To test for equality of variance, Bartlett's test (Hald, 1952) was applied. In summary, this test is based on the principle that the sum of the ratios of individual treatment-group variances to overall combined variance (i.e., all treatment groups) has a X^2 distribution. The null hypothesis asserts that the population variances of the three treatments are equal, and that the observed sample variances are due to the sampling process. The level of significance was set to 1 percent (p=0.01). With 2 degrees of freedom in this comparison, a 1 percent level of significance means that the null hypothesis can be refuted if the computed X^2 value is greater than 9.21.

Table 6 lists X^2 values found using Bartlett's test on the response time data. It is shown that, for the brake and motor failures, the differences in observed variances are statistically significant at the 1 percent level, leading to the conclusion that the population variances are not equal. Although Hald (1952) describes further quantitative tests used to identify individual treatments, which differ significantly. These tests are designed for experiments with a large number of treatments and are not well suited for a three-treatment experiment. However, inspecting variance statistics leads us to the qualitative conclusion that, in both the brake and motor failure data, the variance of the partial automation treatment far exceeds the other two treatments. Thus, we can conclude that the use of partial automation leads to a change in the visual attention bias of the engineer from in-cab monitoring to environment monitoring, and the use of partial automation therefore has a negative impact on the consistency of response to unexpected brake and motor failures because the visual attention of the engineer is biased away from the instrument panel.

With obstruction data, Bartlett's test showed there was no significant difference between the sample variances of the three treatments. Thus, we can conclude that the population variances of the three treatments are equal, and sample variances can be combined to estimate the population variance used in the ANOVA.

Table 6. Results of Bartlett's Test

	Brake Failure	Motor Failure	Obstruction
X^2 value	12.5	24.3	1.1

A one-way ANOVA was performed on the obstruction data to identify the significance of differences in observed mean response times. In this test, the null hypothesis states that the population means are equal. A significance level of 5 percent (p=0.05) was used. With values of 2 and 69 for the degrees of freedom, the null hypothesis can be refuted if the computed F statistic exceeds a value of 3.13.

In the case of the obstruction data, the resulting F statistic from the ANOVA was calculated to be equal to 0.4415. Since this value does not exceed the 5 percent significance value of 3.13, the null hypothesis cannot be refuted—there was no difference, at the 5 percent significance level, between the three levels of automation when comparing mean response time to the obstruction failure. Therefore, we can conclude that varying the automation level has no effect on response time when the engineer is presented with an unexpected obstruction.

3.2 Response Accuracy

In addition to the response time measures, subject response to failure events was evaluated with respect to response accuracy. This evaluation focused on determining whether the engineer's first response was correct for the failure that had occurred.

For each failure scenario, there was a prescribed response pattern. This response was specified in the tutorial material, and practiced during the training sessions. Based on the training, a *correct* response was judged as one in which the subject followed the procedure. A *mistake* occurred when a subject response included an action, which was not part of the prescribed procedure, but was not judged to have a high level of risk to either the passengers or the machinery. An example of a mistake is the depression of the wrong circuit breaker reset button when a motor failure has occurred. A *serious error* is defined as a subject action, which might have a high level of risk to either the passengers or the machinery. An example of a serious error is opening the passenger doors while the vehicle is moving.

Prior to the experimental tests, each subject experienced each failure at least five times, in both expected and unexpected scenarios (Section 2.4.1). Based on the subject responses to the failures during the training sessions, it was observed that they were sufficiently trained in the response procedures to allow adequate response when the failures occurred unexpectedly.

As shown in Tables 7 through 9, very few mistakes occurred, and even fewer serious errors occurred. Table 7 shows the response accuracy data for the brake failures; Table 8 shows the response accuracy data for the motor failures; Table 9 contains the response accuracy data for the obstruction failures. In all cases, the total number of opportunities for mistakes and serious errors is 24—each failure occurrence represents an opportunity for inaccurate response. Tables 7 through 9 contain the total number of inaccurate responses per treatment and error category, as well as the computed error percentages.

Table 7. Summary of Brake Failure Response Accuracy

	Manual		Partial		Full	
	N	%	N	%	N	%
Mistakes	1	4.2	2	8.3	0	0.0
Serious Errors	0	0.0	0	0.0	0	0.0

Table 8. Summary of Motor Failure Response Accuracy

	Manual		Partial		Full	
	N	%	N	%	N	%
Mistakes	2	8.3	2	8.3	2	8.3
Serious Errors	0	0.0	1	4.2	0	0.0

Table 9. Summary of Obstruction Failure Response Accuracy

	Manual		Partial		Full	
	N	%	N	%	N	%
Mistakes	0	0.0	0	0.0	0	0.0
Serious Errors	0	0.0	0	0.0	1	4.2

The best statistical analysis for comparing these data is an X^2 goodness-of-fit test (Hamburg and Young, 1994). The goal was to determine whether the occurrence of operator error differs significantly in any of the test treatments. If there were no difference among the treatments, the percentage of error would be equal across all three treatments for each failure type and seriousness level. Thus, the null hypothesis states that the distribution of failure occurrence is uniform among the three levels of automation. An X^2 value was calculated for each category of accuracy data (three types of failures, each having two levels of accuracy). The expected value is estimated from the observed data, the number of degrees of freedom in each test is therefore equal to one. At a significance level of 5 percent (p=0.05), the resultant X^2 value must exceed 3.84 in order to refute the null hypothesis and conclude that there are significant differences in the observed response accuracy. In all cases, the calculated X^2 value was substantially less than the decision threshold shown in Table 10. As a result, it was concluded that there is no significant difference in response accuracy between the treatments. This conclusion holds across all three failure types.

Table 10. Computed X2 Values for Response Accuracy

Test	X^2 Value
Brake Failure, Mistake	0.667
Brake Failure, Serious Error	0.000
Motor Failure, Mistake	0.000
Motor Failure, Serious Error	0.667
Obstruction, Mistake	0.000
Obstruction, Serious Error	0.667

It is important to interpret these results in context. Determining the response error data poses great difficulty, as a result of the difficulty inherent in differentiating between an incorrect response to a perceived failure versus an incidental action in absence of failure perception. The major difficulty lies in the lack of a method for determining whether the subject actually perceives the failure. In light of this difficulty, the response accuracy results lead to limited conclusions. In addition, the subjects' performance displayed a ceiling effect, in that there were too few errors to detect any differences between the treatments.

3.3 Subjective Evaluation

After the final test session, each subject completed an exit questionnaire (Appendix D), which requested subjective opinions about the correlation between situation awareness and supervisory control. The questionnaire also asked the subjects to rank their preferences. Tabulated results appear in Table 11. The data in Table 11 includes responses from the 12 subjects that completed the full sequence of tests.

Table 11. Subjective Situation Awareness Evaluation and Preference

	Awareness			Preference		
	High	Medium	Low	High	Medium	Low
Manual	9	3	0	3	4	5
Partial	3	6	3	3	5	4
Full	0	3	9	6	3	3

There is a negative correlation between the degree of automation and the perceived situation awareness (i.e., most of the subjects correlated the highest relative level of awareness with manual control and the lowest relative level of awareness with full automation).[2] However, Table 11 also shows that there is no clear correlation between preference and automation level. This indicates that, despite their perception of a degrading effect of supervisory control on operator awareness, some subjects still prefer to use the supervisory control. This leads to the belief that the individual decision to use supervisory control systems was determined by a more complex set of criteria than the perception of awareness.

In addition to eliciting subject preferences, the exit questionnaire contained a section for additional comments. These, along with informal comments during the tests, led to some conclusions, which were not exposed objectively by the experiment. With regard to task workload, the subjects generally felt underutilized. Even in the highest workload case (i.e., manual control), subjects indicated that the overall task was fairly boring. (One subject joked about naming the wayside objects to alleviate the boredom.) It was also evident that the period of highest workload was during station-stopping maneuvers.

With regard to the programmed stop functionality, it was generally agreed that programmed stop was a valuable addition. The consistency in station stopping provided by programmed stop (and by the autopilot, by association) was roundly appreciated. However, as a result of the payoff from the bonus system, some subjects would have preferred to use manual control to achieve more accurate stopping performance, at the risk of consistency, if they had been allowed to choose. It is not clear that such a preference would exist in the absence of a bonus system.

---

[2] There is difficulty using detailed statistical analysis on this type of data because of the subjective nature of the question and response. One possible approach is to assign values to each level (e.g., "high"=3, "medium"=2, and "low"=1), then tally up and compare the results. Using these numbers, it could be concluded that subjective situation awareness strongly favored manual control (with a score of 33, versus 24 for partial automation, and 15 for full automation), while the subject preferences show a slight favor of full automation (with a score of 27, versus 23 for partial automation and 22 for manual control). However, the assignment of numerical values to the ordinal rating is arbitrary, and a little number manipulation could alter those results. Thus, the authors are hesitant to use detailed analysis for this purpose.

4. DISCUSSION AND INTERPRETATION

The results suggest that certain types of supervisory control do impact locomotive engineers' performance in high-speed rail systems. Of the three automation levels used by the subjects, partial automation (cruise control, in particular) led to a higher level of variability in response time to brake and motor failures. This effect was not observed with respect to grade crossing obstructions. Failure response accuracy did not show any significant differences in performance across the three automation treatments. This relationship held true for all three of the failure types experienced by the subjects.

Based on the quantitative results, in combination with qualitative input from the subjects after completion of the experiment, observed effects are believed to be due to differences in attention allocation between automation levels. In all of the attention allocation models presented in Section 1, the capacity for human attention is considered a finite resource. The attention allocation models describe different theories regarding the division or partitioning of this limited resource.

With rail vehicle operation, the task required substantial monitoring. The engineer was required to monitor the instruments in order to perform speed and position control, the primary task in rail operation. In addition, the engineer was required to monitor the vehicle systems status displays, to detect a vehicle-based failure or emergency that might require immediate action. Finally, the engineer was required to observe and monitor the wayside, in order to identify the position of the vehicle and detect any emergency situations that might require action.

During vehicle operation, the engineer dynamically allocated limited available attention resources. The monitoring task, perceived as "most important" presumably, was allocated the highest proportion of attention. The task identified as "most important" varied as the vehicle proceeded through the system.

At higher levels of supervisory control, engineer monitoring requirements changed. The monitoring load was highest using manual control. The engineer was required to monitor the speed and position displays on the instrument panel, as well as the wayside and the vehicle system status displays. However, because the primary task was speed and position control, attention allocation was biased toward monitoring the speed and position instruments.

With partial automation, the requirement for monitoring the speed and position instruments was relieved. However, the engineer was still required to identify the positions along the route requiring active control. For example, with cruise control, the wayside had to be monitored in order to identify points at which the cruise control could be engaged or disengaged, or points at which the speed setting of the cruise control should be altered. (Because of the high vehicle mass, the response to control inputs is slow. As a result, the engineers tended to use manual control for gross speed changes, and use the cruise control speed modulation for fine tuning of the set speed.) In this operational scenario, the "most important" attention item was the position of the vehicle along the route, and a sizable portion of the available attention monitored the wayside and maintained awareness of vehicle position.

In the full automation mode, the requirement for monitoring the wayside was relieved. Although it was still important for the engineer to maintain an awareness of the vehicle position, the autopilot now had to identify speed change waypoints along the route and control the vehicle speed accordingly. The locomotive engineer's role had been altered to one, more accurately described as supervisory. In this scenario, the "most important" task became failure and emergency situation identification.

It is important to consider the impact of the seriousness of the emergency. The experimental results show the diminishing effects of supervisory control in the grade crossing obstruction emergency, as compared to the brake and motor failures. (There were no significant differences in emergency response performance for the grade crossing obstruction among the three treatment groups.) Because the response time results in the partial automation mode indicate that the attention of the engineer was biased toward the external environment, one might expect the response time data for the grade crossing to be shorter in the partial automation case than the other two scenarios. With no significant difference found in the response time to the grade crossing obstruction implies that the subjects perceived the grade crossing obstruction to be a more serious emergency, and therefore allocated more attention to detection of this condition. It is also noteworthy that the grade crossing obstruction could occur only at a few known points on the track. Knowing about the potential emergency, subjects may have paid greater attention to the grade crossings as they approached them, decreasing the likelihood of differences in the response times to obstructions.

5. CONCLUSIONS AND RECOMMENDATIONS

In summary, we can draw the following conclusions:

1. Certain types of supervisory control had a significant effect on variance in response times to the brake and motor failures. In both types of failure, the highest variance was observed with partial automation (i.e., the engineer used the cruise-control and programmed-stop systems). Increase in response time variance can be an indication of an operator out-of-the-loop condition, suggesting degraded situation awareness on the part of the locomotive engineer.

2. Different levels of supervisory control had no significant effect on the response time to the grade crossing obstruction failures, suggesting that engineers were equally attentive to risks in the grade crossings, despite the level of supervisory control. Because the grade crossings occurred at fixed locations, the opportunities for grade crossing obstruction occurred at those known fixed points. This suggests that it might be easier for engineers to prepare for obstruction response than for brake and motor failures, which could occur at any point along the travel route.

3. The response accuracy data, for all failure types, imply that no significant differences in response accuracy exist as a result of using supervisory control. However, this analysis is limited by the quantity of data obtained in the experiment. The occurrence of such errors may be rare enough that true estimates of the relative error rate could not be obtained with the limited number of data points. Expanding the experiment to better capture these effects was beyond the scope of this experiment.

4. The subjective preference data indicate that the subjects perceived a difference in their own situation awareness between the presented levels of supervisory control. Specifically, the subjects felt that increasing the level of supervisory control led to a degradation in awareness. Despite this trend, some subjects preferred to use the automation, leading to the conclusion that the selection of automation level is governed by additional factors.

Based on these conclusions, we can also draw some additional inferences about the effects of supervisory control. Observed differences in behavior were related to the nature of the vehicle speed control loop and shifts in attention resources. In manual mode, the primary task of the locomotive engineer was speed regulation, and the engineer made heavy use of the instruments to perform the task. Although the engineer also observed the wayside for position fixes, braking points, and potential obstructions in grade crossings, the attention allocation was biased toward the instruments. When cruise-control operation was invoked, speed regulation was relaxed. When using cruise control, the engineer was relieved from the lower level control loop, and a greater portion of operator attention was available for greater concentration on the wayside for observance of braking points and other pertinent information. In the process, less attention was directed toward the instrument panel, leading to a higher variability in response time to failures that are detected via the instrument panel. In autopilot mode, the need to observe the wayside was relaxed, as braking points were automatically monitored by the autopilot. The operator could then redirect the available attention resources toward monitoring the instrument panel.

Despite the time spent by each subject, it is believed that performance effects due to complacency were not observed. Although 15 hours per subject is a substantial level of participation, it does not nearly approach the level required to induce complacency and boredom.

Advantages of supervisory control include performance consistency. In general, when comparing automatic control against human control, automatic control provides better performance with regard to consistent and accurate behavior in routine tasks, while the human controller is better suited to adaptation under unexpected circumstances. These characteristics hold true in rail operation. The automatic control systems in the high-speed rail simulator provided tightly maintained speed control (cruise control), consistent station stopping performance (programmed stop), and accurate tracking of pre-determined speed trajectories (autopilot).

However, when considering the overall human-machine system performance, it was observed that the use of cruise control led to a higher variability in the human response to certain emergency situations, thereby offsetting the consistency that had been gained through use of the automatic system. The overall system performance, relative to the specific failures tested, was in fact degraded by this partial automation when compared to the fully manual scenario.

Implementing full automation would be useful in high-speed rail systems. Full automation (autopilot) provides advantages in stopping and schedule consistency, and the overall safety-related performance of the vehicle operators was not degraded when compared to the fully manual control scenario. Full automation use freed sufficient attention resources to maintain or improve response to vehicle-related failures, without significant degradation in response to wayside-related failures.

However, there is concern regarding potential effects of complacency and boredom of incorporating a fully automatic vehicle control system for high-speed rail systems. Although degradation of emergency performance in wayside-related failures was not observed in the short-term, it is not clear that such performance would be maintained over longer-term operating periods. The subjective assessment that situation awareness is degraded when using full automation provides cause to suspect the potential for longer-term effects. Additional research should be conducted to further explore the effects of supervisory control on operator complacency.

The experimental results also raise concerns with regard to safety-related system performance in using cruise control in high-speed rail systems. Cruise control use seems to bias the operator's visual attention away from the in-cab instruments and toward the external environment. This is a benefit in the traditional automotive application of cruise control as attention to the environment results in improved vehicle control performance in dense and highly dynamic traffic. However, in the high-speed rail application, a high percentage of the operator's attention should be focused on monitoring the vehicle systems, and the use of cruise control degrades performance of the operator with regard to vehicle systems monitoring. Because the operator's visual attention is directed out of the cab, the operator performance relative to grade crossing safety was not compromised to any significant degree.

It is possible that the use of a head-up display (HUD), in conjunction with cruise control, might ameliorate the effects of the attention bias induced by the cruise control. A properly designed

HUD would display the pertinent systems state information in the line of sight of the operator when looking out the windshield toward the environment. Having these data in the direct field of view would potentially result in faster response times to systems failures (assuming that the HUD provides a detectable indication of the system failures). It is suggested that a follow-up experiment be conducted to evaluate the changes in operator performance that result from the use of an HUD in conjunction with cruise control.

APPENDIX A. TRAINING TUTORIAL

This appendix presents the written tutorial document, provided to all of the candidate subjects prior to the first training session in the simulation system. The tutorial appears exactly as presented to the test subjects, with the exception that the reference numbers for the figures and tables have been altered to reflect their location in this report (for the purpose of clarifying references to the figures from other sections of the report).

Experiment — General

You are participating in an experiment which will answer questions about the relationship between control automation and operator situation awareness in high-speed rail operation. Although the control of rail vehicles and systems can be automated, there are concerns about potential side effects when using automated control in high-speed rail systems. In order to explore these effects, test subjects like yourself are asked to operate a simulated high-speed train in a virtual reality environment. Your actions are measured during the tests, and later analyzed.

Participation in the experiment consists of two phases. The first phase is a period of training, which consists of a 3-hour instruction session and a 3-hour practice session. Prior to the instruction session, you are asked to review this document, which is a tutorial on the operation of the simulated train vehicle. At the start of the instruction session, you will take a written review quiz, which will gauge your understanding of this material. The written review quiz consists of 25 multiple-choice questions, and is closed book. The quiz is graded immediately after completion. You will then be directed by the instructor through a set of training instructions, which will familiarize you with normal operation of the vehicle. You will also be exposed to a set of emergency scenarios, allowing you to learn the proper responses to these situations.

The second half of the training phase consists of a combination practice and test session. This session is conducted like a regular experiment session, in that it is a 3-hour session consisting of three round trips between the two stations in the system. The first hour is considered to be the practice portion. During this period, you will reacquaint yourself with the operation of the train simulator. The remaining 2 hours is considered a "road test" which will further gauge your abilities to operate the train. Your performance with regard to speed compliance, signal compliance, and station stopping accuracy will be evaluated. If you pass this test, you will be ready ("certified") to perform the experiment trials. You will be eligible for payment for the training phase upon completion of the practice and test session.

The second phase consists of a set of experiment trials. These experiment trials will take place in three separate 3-hour sessions. Each session is called a **shift**, and corresponds to a shift of operation in an actual rail operation. During each shift, you will operate the simulated vehicle as if it were part of an actual rail system. Once underway, you will be expected to remain at the simulator controls ("in the vehicle") until the shift is complete. Brief break periods are allowed, as approved by the experimenter (acting as the CTC operator [and also called the train dispatcher]). The three experiment trials will be conducted on 3 separate days. You will be eligible for payment for the experiment trials upon completion of the third shift.

Payment for the experiment is through the MIT voucher payroll system. The rate of pay is $25 per 3-hour session. Therefore, the subtotal for the training phase is $50, and the subtotal for the experiment phase is $75, resulting in a total payment of $125. (Payment for the experiment phase is subject to performance bonuses, as well as penalties that result from illegal behavior—please refer to the section titled "System Operation — Operator Performance Requirements" for details.) Subjects are paid for each phase completed, regardless of performance. However, subjects that do not pass the training phase will not be allowed to continue with the experimental phase. Subjects can elect payment for the training and experimental phases to be separate (resulting in two checks), or payment for the two phases can be lumped together into one check.

This tutorial is organized so that the reader can learn the fundamentals of rail system operation in a logical order. Important terms and concepts are highlighted with bold-faced text.

System Operation — General

The rail system used in the experiment is a fictitious rail system connecting two stations, named West Station and East Station (Figure A-1). The two stations are connected via a single track that is 31 miles (50 km) in length. At each end of system, beyond the stations, there is a loop of track that is used to turn the vehicles around for the return trip.

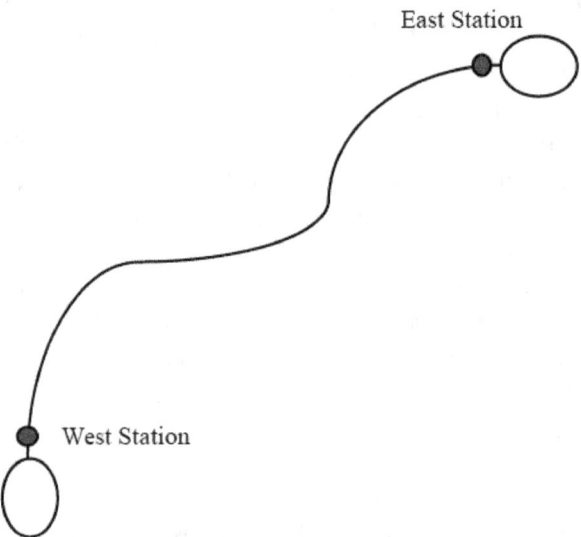

Figure A-1. Track Layout, Simulated Rail System

The system is operated as a high-speed shuttle between these two stations. There is one vehicle in operation. That vehicle will travel from one station to the other, discharge passengers, loop around to reverse direction, board new passengers, and proceed to the other station. This procedure is followed throughout the duration of the shift.

Operation of the system is coordinated through a **central traffic control** operator (**CTC**). This person is located in a fixed position in the system, and has access to the state of all the vehicles operating in the system. The CTC operator has the task of coordinating the operation of several vehicles that must share resources (such as the track system). To carry this task out, the CTC operator has control over the switches in the system, and can set signal levels manually. In addition, the CTC operator is able to communicate directly with vehicle operators.

The **wayside** is a general term which refers to all objects in the environment which do not move. This includes items such as the ground, the track, the signal lights, the surrounding trees and buildings, and so on.

System Operation — Block Signal System

Rail systems have traditionally used a system known as **block signaling** for control of trains in the rail system. With block signaling, the track is divided into fixed length chunks known as **blocks**. While the length of each block does not change, different blocks are not necessarily of equal length. Typically, shorter block lengths are used in the near vicinity of stations, while longer block lengths are used in regions away from the stations. Block lengths are generally on the order of one mile. In the road system used in the simulation, all blocks between stations are 1.2 miles (2 km), and all blocks in the loop sections are 0.6 miles (1 km) in length.

At the boundaries of each block is a **signal light**. This signal light displays a color-coded signal, which indicates the maximum speed permitted throughout the block. The signal acts as a dynamic **speed limit**, and it is the responsibility of the vehicle operator to identify the signal as the block boundary is approached and set the vehicle speed accordingly.

A fundamental rule in block signaling is that no more than one train can occupy a block at any given time. A red signal is used to indicate that another train currently occupies the block, and the approaching train is not permitted to enter that block. The blocks that precede the occupied block have signal levels which ensure that the train can be slowed in time to stop before entering the occupied block.

In addition to the speed limits imposed by the block signal system, there are also **civil speed limits**, which are static. These limits are either memorized or written down by the operator. In all cases, the prevailing speed limit is the lesser of the block signal limit and the civil speed limit.

The exact specification of signals used and speed limits associated with those signals is a design parameter for a rail system, and varies from system to system. In the simulation system, a five-aspect signaling system is used. This means that there are five color codes used in the system, with the codes defined as shown in Table A-1.

If a train was occupying block 157, then the signal at the entrance to block 157 would show STOP (red), the signal at the entrance to block 156 would show RESTRICTED (red/yellow), the signal at the entrance to block 155 would show APPROACH (yellow), the signal at the entrance to block 154 would show APPROACH MEDIUM (green/yellow), and the signals at blocks prior to 154 would show CLEAR (green). The speed limits apply to the entire block, which means an approaching train must reduce speed to the limit before reaching the entrance of the block. So, in this example scenario, another train approaching the train in block 157 must be going slower than 143 mph (230 km/h) before entering block 154, slower than 93 mph (150 km/h) before entering block 155, and slower than 50 mph (80 km/h) before entering block 156 (see Figure A-2).

Table A-1. Rail Signal Codes

COLOR	CODE	ACTION
Red	STOP	not permitted to enter the block
red/yellow	RESTRICTED	maximum speed of 50 mph (80 km/h) in this block
Yellow	APPROACH	maximum speed of 93 mph (150 km/h) in this block
green/yellow	APPROACH MEDIUM	maximum speed of 143 mph (230 km/h) in this block
Green	CLEAR	maximum speed of 186 mph (300 km/h) in this block

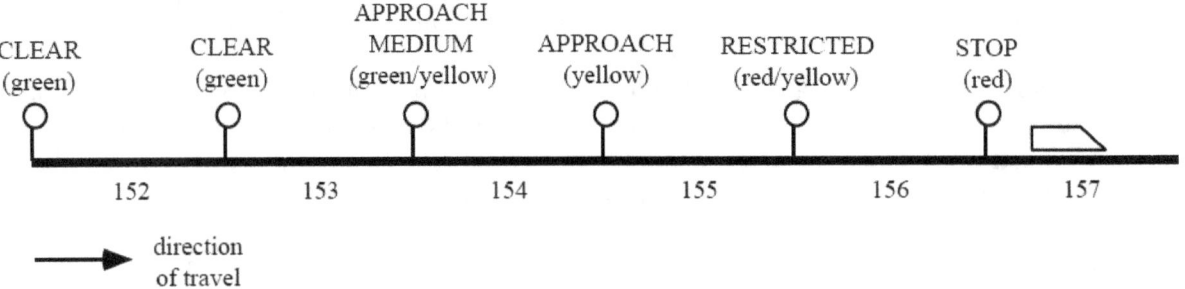

Figure A-2. Block Signaling System

Located throughout the system are position markers known as **mileposts**. The use of these by vehicle operators is discussed in detail in the next section. It is important to note the difference between block signals and mileposts. At the entrance to each block, there is a signal board which identifies the block number and displays the current signal level for that block. Because block boundaries occur at 1.2 mi (2 km) intervals on the main line in this system, there is also typically a milepost at the block boundaries. So, for example, block 13 comprises the distance of track between mileposts 26 and 28. This provides opportunity for confusion: When traveling eastbound, the entrance to block 13 is marked by mile post 26, but when traveling westbound, the entrance to the same block occurs at mile post 28. Operators must take care to differentiate between block identifiers and mileposts, as the relationship between them is not as simple as it might at first appear.

Vehicle Operation — User Interface

The user interface for the train simulation consists of two graphics displays, a computer keyboard, and the combined control lever. The two graphics displays are placed side by side on a table, with the computer keyboard between them and the combined control lever to the right.

The display to the right is the instrument panel for the train. A schematic drawing of the instrument layout is shown in Figure A-3. In this figure, we can locate the speedometer, the secondary gauges (brake tank pressure, wheel bearing temperature, and trolley voltage), the mode indicators, the warning indicators, the motor current meters, the system clock, and the communications display.

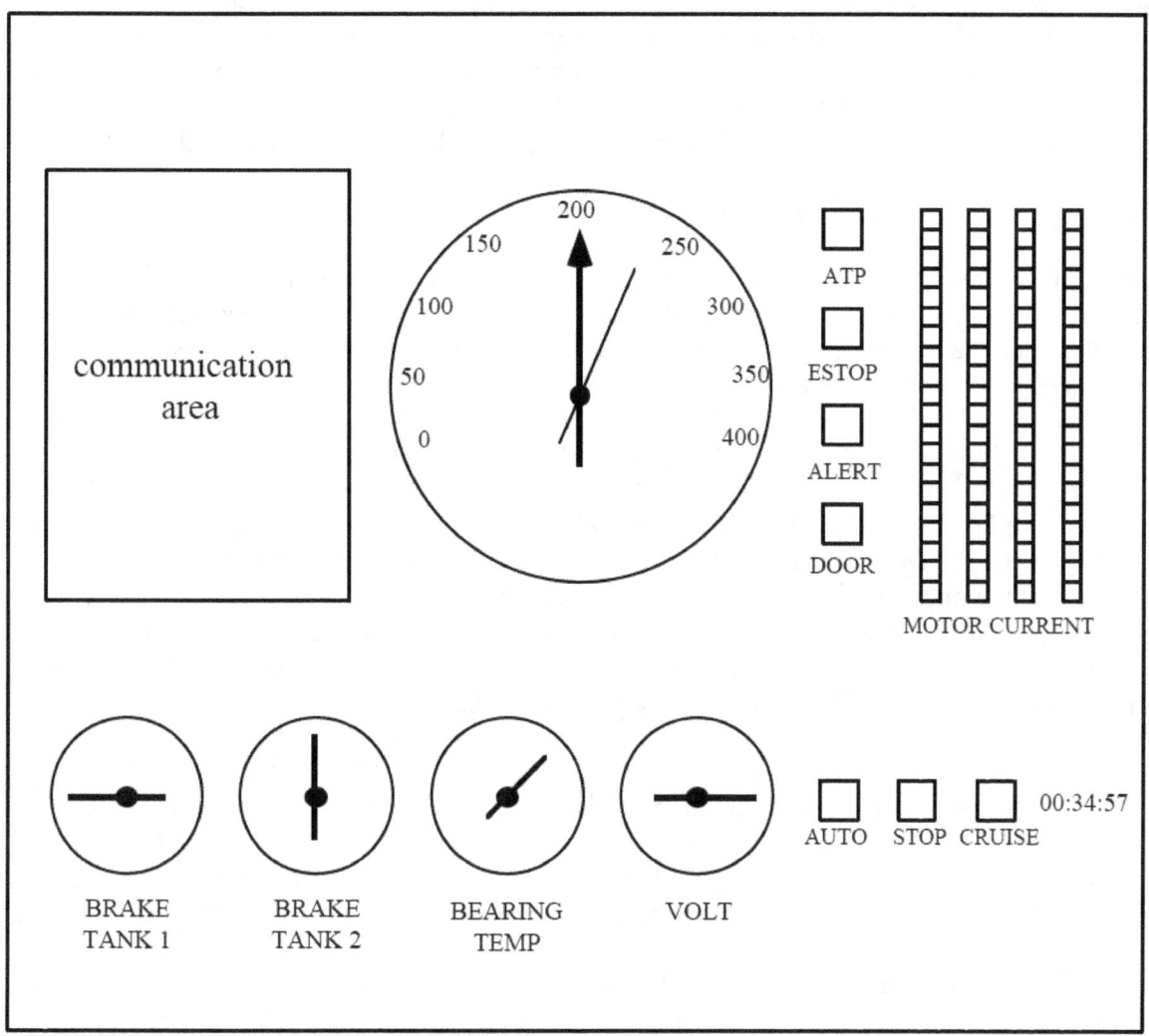

Figure A-3. Instrument Panel Layout

The graphics display on the left is the out-the-window view port. This is also known as the **windscreen**. In this view, the operator is able to view the world outside the vehicle. The scene presented is a night scene, with wire-frame objects along the wayside. This port also provides a head-up display for assistance in station stopping (described in a later section), as well as an indication of collision with a highway vehicle in a grade crossing (described in a later section).

The **combination control lever** is a joystick-like lever to the right of the keyboard (beside the instrument panel display). Although there are two handles on the control, only the right black-handled lever is used. This lever is used to control both the thrust and braking commands, with the forward (up) direction for thrust and the backward (down) direction for braking. The center position (coast) is notched for reference.

The computer keyboard is used for both control buttons and alphanumeric communications input. The function buttons in the top row have specific operator control functions, described in

35

the following sections. The main part of the keyboard is for entry of communications messages. These messages are typed in, and are displayed in the communications area of the instrument panel. While a message is being composed, it appears in the lower portion of the communications display, and is visible to only the operator. When the carriage return is depressed, the message is "sent" to all other operators on the system, including the CTC operator. The message then appears in the "receive" area (top portion) of the communications display. The messages that appear in the top portion are visible to all operators in the system.

Vehicle Operation — Head-Up Display for Station Stopping

Because of the braking dynamics of rail trains, one of the more challenging aspects of train operation is stopping the vehicle at an appropriate point in the station. This becomes very important when the vehicle must be stopped at a precise point, for example, to allow proper alignment of handicapped ramps.

Because of the limited perspective through the out-the-window viewport, a decision aid is provided in the train simulator to assist the vehicle operator in this task. The aid takes the form of a **head-up display** (or HUD), which is a graphical icon superimposed on the windscreen. (Head-up displays are commonly found in military aircraft, where a set of instrument displays is projected on the windscreen so that the pilots can monitor the vehicle status while concurrently performing other visual tasks.) The HUD in the train is a yellow rectangular box, which appears when the train is within the confines of the station. When the HUD is aligned with the back wall of the station, the train is at the ideal stopping point in the station.

In the event that the vehicle comes to a stop before it is in the station (i.e., before the HUD appears), the operator can slowly bring the vehicle into the appropriate position. If the vehicle comes to a stop after the station is passed (overshoot), the operator must contact the CTC to report the situation and request further instruction. Under no circumstances should the vehicle operator open the passenger doors if the vehicle is not within the boundaries of the station.

Vehicle Operation — Speed and Position Control

The most important task required of a train vehicle operator is the control of vehicle speed. The operator uses the position of the vehicle to obtain the current speed limit, through a combination of civil speed limits (which are memorized or written down) and block signal states (which are observed on the wayside). The operator then uses the traction motor system and the braking system to adjust the speed of the vehicle accordingly.

The vehicle operator gets information about vehicle speed through the speedometer, which is located on the instrument panel in the locomotive cab. In the train simulation, this speedometer is implemented as a round dial gauge. The units shown are kilometers per hour (km/h), and the available range of speeds is from 0 to 217.5 mph (350 km/h). The major increments of the gauge display are 31.1 mph (50 km/h), with minor increments each 6.2 mph (10 km/h). The red pointer indicates the current speed, while the smaller yellow pointer (underneath the red pointer) indicates the set speed (used by the automation systems).

Another important task of the vehicle operator is monitoring the position of the vehicle in the rail system. Monitoring the out-the-window view accomplishes this. Along the wayside, distance is marked through the use of "mile posts." Typically, at one-mile intervals, a post is placed on the wayside with numbers indicating the mile marker. Vehicle operators use the difference between posts to measure distances along the road. Because the simulation system is implemented using the metric system, these posts are referred to as "mile posts," and are located at one-kilometer intervals.

When approaching a stopping point, such as a station, the vehicle operator uses out-the-window cues to identify points at which the brakes should be applied to stop at a particular position. Because of the high mass of the train (with resultant high momentum when in motion), accurately braking the vehicle requires relatively long lead times for the control commands. As a result, it is common for train operators in real systems to use stationary objects on the wayside as braking point markers. Learning the proper braking points represents a significant part of the training process for vehicle operators.

To assist in learning and remembering the appropriate braking points, there are significant landmarks placed in the wayside environment at points that help locate the braking points. During the training phase, the subject is provided with a three-page chart titled "Brake Point Specification Worksheet." This worksheet shows a schematic diagram of the track, and identifies the speed restricted areas, as well as the braking points for these areas. The chart also identifies the landmarks which are placed near each braking point.

Blocks 0, 1, 11, 12, and 13 all have speed restrictions, due to the grade crossings present in these blocks. When traveling from West Station to East Station, the first major braking point occurs at milepost 17, to slow from 186 mph (300 km/h) to 62 mph (100 km/h) before reaching block 11. At 17, on the right, there is a group of 5 red columns that serve as a landmark. The next major braking point is at milepost 44, for stopping at East Station. The landmark at this point is a large red building on the left, surrounded by a blue fence. When traveling from East Station to West Station, the first braking point occurs at milepost 33, to slow in time for the speed restriction at block 13. In this case, the landmark is a red pedestrian bridge over the track. Finally, at milepost 9, there is a large red building with a green pointed crown on its roof, located to the left side, signifying the braking point for entrance to block 1. These landmarks are noted on the Brake Point Specification Worksheet.

The skill of stopping the train at the station is a critical component of vehicle operation in passenger rail systems. Tables A-2 and A-3 are provided to assist in learning this skill. In the simulation system, the ideal stopping point in the station is defined as the point at which the front of the train is just underneath the block signal sign. As described in the previous section ("Vehicle Operation — Head-Up Display for Station Stopping"), there is a decision aid to assist in locating this position. Table A-2 is a summary of the relationship between the position in the station and the visual cues in the out-the-window view. Table A-3 provides a summary of the braking distances from low speed, using full service braking. From the information provided in these tables, the following strategy for accurate station stopping can be determined:

1) Enter the station at about 21.7 mph (35 km/h).

2) Apply full service braking as the vehicle passes through the entrance doorway.

3) When the vehicle slows to 6.2 mph (10 km/h), ease off the brakes to coast.

4) When the middle of the block signal sign intersects the top of the windscreen, re-apply full service braking.

In addition, Table A-3 shows that entrance to the station at a speed in excess of 24.9 mph (40 km/h) will result in overshoot, and may result in a missed station stop.

Vehicle Operation — Control Modes

There are four basic **control modes** available with the high-speed rail simulation vehicle: a) manual mode, b) cruise control mode, c) programmed stop mode, and d) autopilot mode. The latter three are considered **automatic control modes** because part of the vehicle control task is performed by a computer-based control system.
In **manual mode**, the vehicle operator is responsible for all aspects of vehicle control. Using the **combination control lever**, the vehicle operator provides all thrust and brake commands required to achieve speed and position control of the vehicle.
In **cruise control mode**, the automatic control system applies the appropriate level of thrust force to maintain a constant speed setting. The vehicle operator is responsible for determining the proper speed for the conditions, and then setting the cruise control system for that speed.

Table A-2. Relationship Between Vehicle Position and Out-the-Window View

Position, relative to stopping point	visual cue
-360.9 ft (-110 m) (undershoot)	entrance doorway is just visible in windscreen
-328 ft (-100 m)	HUD (yellow rectangle) appears on windscreen
-180.4 ft (-55 m)	HUD top bar at top of block signal sign
-180.4 ft (-40 m)	HUD top bar across middle of block sign
-91.8 ft (-28 m)	HUD top bar at bottom of block sign
-65.6 ft) (-20 m)	HUD top bar midway between bottom of block sign and top of back wall
-39.4 ft (-12 m)	top of block sign at top of windscreen
-29.5 ft (-9 m)	middle of block sign at top of windscreen
-19.7 ft (-6 m)	bottom of block sign at top of windscreen
0	HUD aligned with back wall
+98.4 ft (+30 m)	top of HUD halfway down upper portion (purple) of back wall
+187 ft (+57 m)	HUD top bar at top of exit doorway
+239.5 ft (+73 m)	HUD side bars at sides of exit doorway
+295.3 ft (+90 m)	exit doorway is just visible in windscreen
+328 ft (+100 m) (overshoot)	HUD display disappears

Table A-3. Summary of Low-Speed Braking Distances

speed (mph)	stopping distance (feet) (FSB)
24.9 (40 km/h)	363 (110 m)
21.7 (35 km/h)	280.5 (85 m)
18.6 (30 km/h)	204.6 (62 m)
15.5 (25 km/h)	145.2 (44 m)
12.4 (20 km/h)	92.4 (28 m)
9.3 (15 km/h)	52.8 (16 m)
6.2 (10 km/h)	26.4 (8 m)
3.1 (5 km/h)	6.6 (2 m)

In **programmed stop mode**, the automatic control system applies the appropriate level of brake force to stop the vehicle at a specific position. The vehicle operator is responsible for determining the appropriate position to invoke the programmed stop mode.

In the **autopilot mode**, the automatic control system applies the appropriate level of thrust and brake forces to follow a predetermined speed trajectory. The vehicle operator is responsible for invoking the autopilot control mode. Once vehicle control has been assumed by the automatic control system, all necessary vehicle control commands are provided by the control system. The task of the operator is reduced to monitoring the vehicle and wayside systems, looking for potential problems in operation.

Vehicle Operation — Traction System

In general, high-speed trains are propelled by electric motors, called **traction motors**. Power for the traction motors is fed from a high-voltage line, usually on overhead wires. The power is then passed through a **motor controller**, which governs the amount of power supplied to the traction motors based on the control command of either the vehicle operator or automatic control system.

In the manual operating mode, the vehicle operator is in direct control of the traction power via the combination control lever. Moving the lever forward increases the level of power, and consequently, the acceleration of the vehicle. When the control lever is in the center position, no tractive power is provided, and the vehicle coasts. Moving the lever back increases the braking force.

In the three automatic modes (autopilot, cruise control, and programmed stop), the level of tractive power is determined automatically by the control system, and a control command is provided to the traction motor controller.

When tractive power is commanded, either manually or automatically, the motor controller provides electrical power to the traction motors. The tractive force provided by the motor is proportional to the current through the motor windings. The dashboard display includes four current meters (**ammeters**), which display the level of current through each of the four traction motors. In manual mode, these displays will respond directly to the input at the combination control lever, while in automatic mode, they provide a mechanism for observing the operation of the automatic systems.

The traction motors are protected by **circuit breakers**, which will interrupt the flow of electrical power to the motors if a failure condition is detected. Each of the four motors has a separate circuit breaker. Under certain circumstances, the circuit breaker for a single traction motor can be tripped, which results in no power being provided to the traction motor. The occurrence of this event can be observed through the ammeters—when one (or more) of the ammeters does not respond with the others, the circuit breaker for that traction motor has tripped and must be reset.

The procedure for resetting the circuit breaker is as follows: a) Remove all power from the other traction motors, by moving the combination control lever to a coast or brake position. b) Depress the appropriate traction motor reset switch (F1 through F4 on the control panel).

c) Apply tractive power manually, using the combination control lever. d) Resume the control mode previously in use. If any of the traction motor reset switches are depressed while power is applied, a safety system causes all of the traction motor circuit breakers to trip, preventing motor overload. In this event, all of the circuit breakers must be reset to resume proper operation.

Vehicle Operation — Brake System

Train brakes utilize air pressure, which is stored in tanks on the locomotive. Under non-braking circumstances, the pressure in the tanks prevents the brakes from engaging. When the brakes are applied, pressure is released from the tanks, causing the brake shoes to contact the rotating surfaces and resulting in a force, which slows the vehicle. An important variable to be monitored by the vehicle operator is the **brake tank pressure.**

The braking system has two separate modes of operation, **service braking** and **emergency braking**. During normal operation, the vehicle operator uses service braking to apply various levels of braking force to the vehicle. In this mode, the combination control lever controls the level of service brake application. The level of braking force can be varied continuously throughout the available range. Application of the maximum available braking force is known as **full service braking.**

In the emergency braking mode, all of the pressure in the brake system is released, resulting in the maximum possible brake force. In general, this is not a desirable event, as the forces generated result in severe deceleration, which can damage equipment and can cause discomfort or injury to passengers. The vehicle operator can command application of the emergency brake via a control switch on the instrument panel. Also, in certain operational modes, the emergency brake will be applied as a result of dangerous conditions or improper control actions. Such application of the emergency brake is known as a **penalty application.**

During application of the emergency brakes, the emergency brake indicator will be lit (red). Once the emergency brakes have been applied, they cannot be released until the vehicle comes to a complete stop. When the vehicle is stopped, the control lever is pulled back to a position that results in application of the service brake, and the emergency brake reset switch is depressed. At that point, the emergency brake indicator light will be extinguished, and the vehicle will be ready to continue with normal operation.

The pressure in the brake tanks is indicated by the brake tank pressure gauges, which are located on the instrument panel. In the train simulation, there are two brake tanks, one each for two separate halves of the brake system. The corresponding gauges are round dial gauges, calibrated in units of pounds per square inch (psi), with a range from 0 to 100 psi. The normal reading when the brakes are not applied (i.e., the nominal high pressure) is approximately 98 psi. When full service braking is applied, the pressure drops to approximately 22 psi, and the pressure further drops to 0 psi under emergency braking.

If there is a failure in the braking system, one or both of the tanks may show a reduction in tank pressure. This situation will result in the brakes being applied without being commanded by either the operator or the control system. The procedure for rectifying this situation is to switch to an alternate brake compressor. This is accomplished by depressing the brake compressor switch (F10 key). The pressure in the faulty tank will then rise to the appropriate level.

Vehicle Operation — Cruise Control Operation

The function of the cruise control system is to maintain a constant vehicle speed. The vehicle operator invokes the cruise control by depressing the cruise control enable switch (F5 key) while the vehicle is traveling at the desired speed.

When the cruise control mode is enabled, the cruise control indicator light (green) is illuminated, and the yellow pointer on the speedometer indicates the set speed. When the cruise control is first selected, the control system will adjust itself to determine the proper level of thrust force required to maintain the selected speed. As a result, there is a small amount of "hunting" around the set speed at first. The system then settles down to the set speed, and small fluctuations in the motor current indicate that the control system is operating.

The vehicle operator can alter the set speed by depressing the "up-arrow" and "down-arrow" keys on the keyboard. With the depression of each key, the set speed is adjusted up (or down) by 0.6 mph (1 km/h). This feature allows the operator to "fine-tune" the set speed. When the operator adjusts the set speed down to a lower speed, the vehicle will coast down to the lower speed.

From cruise control mode, the vehicle operator can either select manual mode or programmed stop mode. By pulling back on the combination control lever, the braking system is actuated, and the vehicle returns to manual mode. The vehicle operator can also directly select programmed stop mode from cruise control mode.

For reasons of safety, application of the brakes will always disengage the cruise control system. As a result, it is not possible to engage the cruise control system when the brakes are in use. If the operator attempts to engage the cruise control system while the brakes are applied, the system will not respond to that mode command, and the vehicle will remain in manual mode.

Vehicle Operation — Programmed Stop Operation

The function of the programmed stop system is to bring the vehicle to a smooth, controlled stop at a predetermined location (specifically, at the end of the currently occupied block). The vehicle operator invokes the programmed stop function by depressing the programmed stop enable switch (F6 key) while the vehicle is traveling at a steady speed that is less than 49.7 mph (80 km/h).

The programmed stop mode must not be invoked when the vehicle is traveling at a speed greater than 49.7 mph (80 km/h). If the vehicle speed is greater than 49.7 mph (80 km/h), activating this mode will result in a penalty application of the emergency brakes. In addition, the programmed stop controller must keep track of the distance between the train and the stopping position (the end of the current block). If the programmed stop mode is invoked while the vehicle is too close to the end of the block to be stopped using full service braking, the emergency brakes will be applied in an attempt to stop the vehicle before the end of the block.

When the programmed mode is enabled, the programmed stop indicator light (orange) is illuminated. The vehicle operator can return to manual mode by pulling back on the combination control lever to activate the braking system.

For reasons of safety, application of the brakes will always disengage the programmed stop control system. As a result, it is not possible to engage the programmed stop mode when the brakes are in use. If the operator attempts to engage programmed stop operation while the brakes are applied, the system will not respond to that mode command, and the vehicle will remain in manual mode.

Vehicle Operation — Autopilot Operation

The function of the autopilot system is to perform all thrust and brake commands required to follow a pre-determined speed trajectory. The vehicle operator invokes the autopilot function by depressing the autopilot enable switch (F7 key) while the vehicle is in motion. For best performance, the vehicle must be traveling at a speed greater than 6.2 mph (10 km/h) when the autopilot is activated.

When the autopilot mode is enabled, the autopilot indicator light (blue) is illuminated. In addition, the yellow pointer on the speedometer indicates the pre-determined speed setting. The vehicle operator can return to manual mode by pulling back on the combination control lever to activate the braking system.

For reasons of safety, application of the brakes will always disengage the autopilot control system. As a result, it is not possible to engage the autopilot mode when the brakes are in use. If the operator attempts to engage the autopilot system while the brakes are applied, the system will not respond to that mode command, and the vehicle will remain in manual mode.

Vehicle Operation — Alerter System

The **alerter system** is a safety system on the train, which reduces the risk of accidents that are due to operator incapacitation or inattention. The principle behind the system is the requirement for periodic input from the vehicle operator, to determine if the operator is still functional at the controls. If the operator does not respond in a reasonable amount of time, the system assumes that the operator is incapacitated, and applies the emergency brakes to stop the vehicle.

The alerter system, as implemented in the high-speed rail simulation, is similar to those used internationally in actual rail systems. If the operator does not depress the alerter response button ("escape" key) within a period of 42 seconds from the last depression of that button, the system issues a warning reminding the operator to do so. The warning consists of a flashing yellow indicator light and an audible chime. If the operator does not respond within 10 seconds of the onset of the warning, the system assumes that the operator is incapacitated and applies the emergency brakes. In this scenario, both the alerter warning light and emergency brake light will be illuminated.

One type of alerter system, known as a **smart alerter**, will acknowledge other command actions by the operator as a response to the alerter system. For example, if the alerter issues a warning and the operator pulls back on the combined control lever to apply the brakes, the alerter system interprets that braking command as a response, and ceases to issue the warning. This type of system presents less of a workload to operators under hectic conditions. The alerter system implemented in the simulation system is a smart alerter system.

Vehicle Operation — ATP System

The **automatic train protection system (ATP)** is a safety system on the train. Its function is to reduce the risk of accident by preventing an overspeed condition to occur. An overspeed condition is defined as operation of the vehicle at speeds in excess of either the civil speed limit or the signal speed limit.

The ATP system continuously monitors the speed and position of the vehicle. It also identifies the state of the block signal when the vehicle enters a block. Based on the position of the vehicle and the block signal state, the maximum allowable speed is determined. If the vehicle exceeds that speed by no more than 9.3 mph (15 km/h), a warning is issued. The warning consists of a flashing yellow indicator light and an audible chime. If the speed is not reduced to a level less than the limit within a period of 20 seconds, or if the speed is greater than 9.3 mph (15 km/h) over the limit, a penalty application of the emergency brakes is invoked. In this scenario, both the ATP warning light and emergency brake light will be illuminated.

Vehicle Operation — Door Control

The vehicle operator is responsible for controlling the state of the **passenger doors**. The doors are to be opened when the vehicle is stopped in the station. In principle, the doors must not be opened at any other point in the system, for the protection of the passengers.

Door control is accomplished through the door control button (F8 button). The door indicator light (red) on the instrument panel shows the state of the doors. When the light is illuminated, the doors are open. Depressing the door control button while the vehicle is stopped will cause the state of the doors to change — if the doors are open, they will be closed, and if the doors are closed, they will be opened.

A safety system prevents the doors from being opened while the vehicle is in motion. Door control commands while the vehicle is in motion will be ignored. If the vehicle is stopped with the doors open, any attempt to move the vehicle will cause a penalty application of the emergency brake.

Vehicle Operation — In-Cab Signal System

In many rail systems using block signal technology, the signal information is available only on the wayside. This type of system presents two distinct problems: the vehicle operator must remember the state of the signal after the vehicle has passed the block boundary, and there is no indication of the signal level of the next block to allow the operator to make preparatory control commands.

Many contemporary locomotive cab designs include **in-cab signals**, which are devices in the cab that display the signal level of the block currently occupied. While this solves the problem of remembering the signal state of the current block, it still does not solve the preview problem.

At true high-speed operation (speeds in excess of 124.3 mph [200 km/h]), it is virtually impossible to see wayside signals in time to take appropriate corrective action. Therefore, such operations require some form of signal preview as part of the in-cab signal system. In the high-speed rail simulation vehicle, the in-cab signal system is implemented with two color-coded light bars, each containing three lights. The bottom light bar displays the color code of the signal state of the currently occupied block when the vehicle entered it. The top light bar displays the color code of the signal state of the next block.

Vehicle Operation — Bearing Temperature Display

One of the secondary gauges provided on the instrument panel of the train simulation displays **wheel bearing temperature**. Train operations have traditionally been concerned about detecting overheated wheel bearings, as an overheated wheel bearing could ultimately seize and lead to derailment. Certain train operations have installed **hot box detectors**, which are wayside-located boxes that detect a hot bearing as the train passes by.

The wheel bearing temperature system in the train simulation uses sensors on each wheel to measure the temperature. The display then shows the temperature of the hottest bearing among those that are measured. In normal operation, the temperature will rise as the speed of the vehicle increases, and fall to ambient temperature when the vehicle slows down. If a wheel bearing does fail, the wheel bearing temperature gauge will reflect the temperature of the hottest bearing. It does not, however, indicate which bearing is at fault—the vehicle operator must stop the train and locate the faulty bearing (usually through observation of smoke at the wheel).

Vehicle Operation — Trolley Voltage Display

One of the secondary gauges in the instrument panel displays the **trolley voltage**, which is the voltage available from the power supply grid to the traction motor controllers (nominally 1500 VDC).

The gauge is provided so that the vehicle operator can detect problems with the power supply voltage, which will have implications on the performance of the vehicle. Although the vehicle operator cannot take any action to rectify such an occurrence, the vehicle operator would be able to inform the CTC operator, via the communication channel, of the problem. The CTC operator would then contact the appropriate personnel in the power supply department in an effort to rectify the problem.

Vehicle Operation — Acceleration and Braking Performance

Although there are many conceptual similarities between operating a rail vehicle and driving an automobile, the biggest difference occurs in braking and acceleration performance. Because of the very large mass of a rail vehicle (typically in the range of hundreds of tons), the distances required for acceleration and braking are much larger than might be expected. This becomes more of an issue as the vehicle speed grows larger—the stopping distances from a speed of 186.4 mph (300 km/h) are on the order of several kilometers.

This situation has several implications. An important safety consideration is that the large stopping distance makes it virtually impossible for an operator to stop in time from high speed for an unexpected track obstruction. The only reasonable solutions to this problem are to reduce the allowable vehicle speeds in risk-prone areas, and to provide additional driving aids, such as obstruction warning systems. In general, operators are not held liable for situations, which are beyond their control.

In the simulation system, this issue is addressed by taking care that there are no unexpected hazards that are beyond the operator's control. Grade crossing areas are the only places where track obstructions can occur. These obstructions take the form of highway vehicles crossing the track. In the grade crossing areas, the civil speed limit is reduced to 62.1 mph (100 km/h). These areas include blocks 0, 1, 11, 12, and 13. Within these areas, the vehicle operator is able to detect and react to an obstruction at a highway grade crossing. Highway vehicles that cross the tracks will only do so when there is sufficient distance for them to clear the crossing before the train arrives. Under certain circumstances, however, the highway vehicle may get stuck at the crossing in the path of the train. By design, the point in time at which the vehicle gets stuck will be such that the train operator has sufficient time to detect the obstruction and stop the train before a collision occurs.

Another implication of large braking distances is the necessity for good judgment of braking points. Because the braking distances are so large, proper planning of braking points is essential for a vehicle to be stopped accurately at stations (or other stopping points). This is a skill, which requires a great deal of practice to master, and represents an important component of operator training programs in actual rail operations. Such training programs typically last for a year or more.

To shorten this learning curve, graphical representations of the vehicle performance curves are shown in Figures A-4 through A-6. Figure A-4 displays the full-throttle acceleration profile on level ground. The speed is shown as a function of distance. From this curve, we can see that the distance required to reach 186.4 mph (300 km/h) from a standing stop is approximately 7.1 mi (11.5 km).

Full Throttle Acceleration Curve

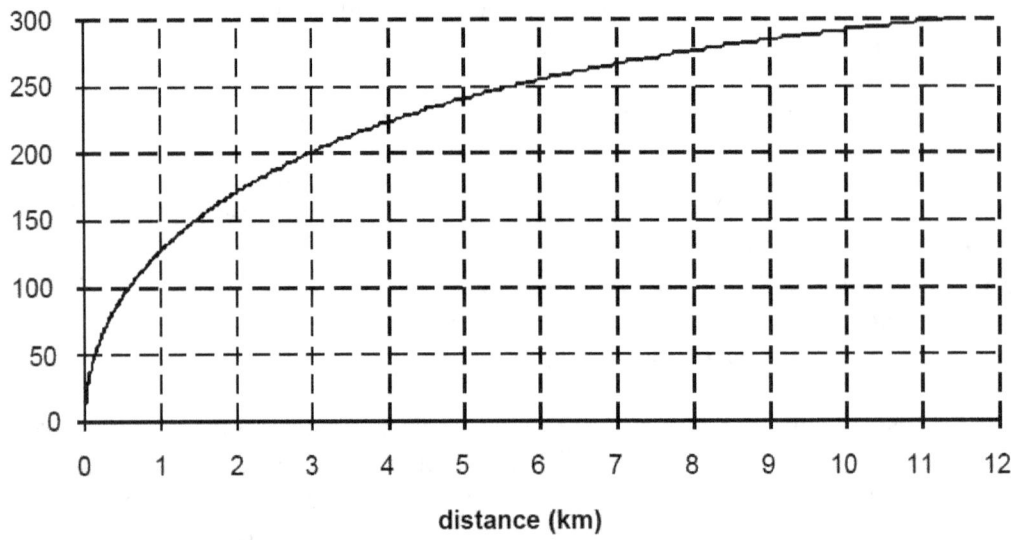

Figure A-4. Full-Throttle Acceleration Profile

In Figure A-5, the full-service braking profile is shown again for the case of travel on level ground. From this curve, we can see that the braking distance from 186.4 mph (300 km/h) is approximately 3.2 mph (5.2 km), which is substantially shorter than the distance required to achieve that speed in the first place (Figure A-4). The reason for this difference is twofold: a) peak braking forces are generally higher than peak traction forces, for safety reasons, and b) at higher speeds, the resultant aerodynamic drag works against acceleration, but contributes to deceleration forces.

Note that the braking distance from 62.1 mph (100 km/h) is just a little larger than a half kilometer. Obstructions in the grade crossings are visible from the vehicle for a distance of almost one kilometer—therefore, this braking performance provides adequate opportunity for the vehicle operator to detect and react properly to an obstruction in a grade crossing.

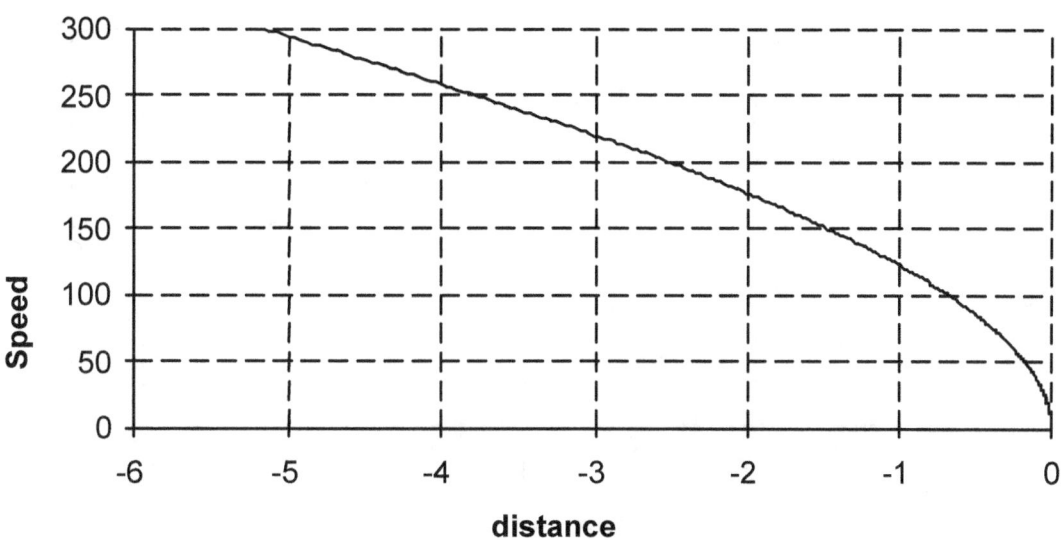

Figure A-5. Full-Service Braking Profile

The full-service braking profile (Figure A-5) can be used to estimate appropriate braking points under manual control. When approaching West Station, there is a civil speed restriction of 62.1 mph (100 km/h) for two blocks (2.5 mi – 4 km) (blocks 0 and 1, which cover the track between mile post 4 and the station) prior to the station, to reduce speed for grade crossing safety. Approaching East Station, there is a similar speed restriction for one block (1.2 mi – 2 km) (block 24, between mile post 48 and the station), to ensure that a train does not go through the station at full speed. In addition, there is a speed-restricted region in blocks 11 through 13 (covering the track between mile posts 22 and 28), for reasons of grade crossing safety. When approaching these regions, full-service braking from full speed (186.4 mph [300 km/h]) should begin 2.8 mi (4.5 km) prior to the start of the restricted block, to ensure that the vehicle speed is at or below the restricted speed before entering that block. When approaching the two stations, the vehicle operator can again apply full service braking in the last block when the vehicle is about 0.6 mi (1 km) from the station, bringing the vehicle to a coasting speed of slightly less than 24.9 mph (40 km/h). As the vehicle passes through the entrance of the station, the vehicle operator can again apply the brakes to stop precisely in the station. The ideal stopping point is the position at which the block signal board is just visible in the windscreen. If the operator stops the vehicle too soon, the vehicle must be brought forward to this point so that the passenger doors may be opened. The operator may legally stop the vehicle forward of this point, as long as the exit doorway and back wall of the station are still visible through the windscreen.

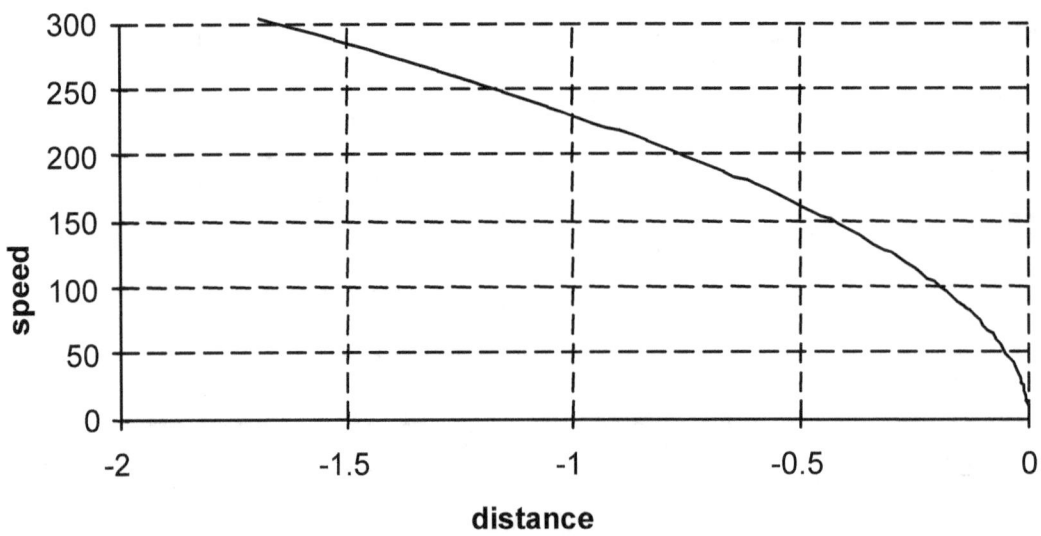

Figure A-6. Emergency Braking Profile

Figure A-6 shows the braking profile under emergency braking conditions. The distance required to brake from 186.4 mph (300 km/h) under emergency stop conditions is only about 1.05 mi (1.7 km). However, this braking performance has a high cost—the more severe deceleration experienced during these stopping conditions is the result of severe forces at the wheels which can result in damaged train equipment, as well as damaged track. In addition, in passenger service, the resultant deceleration can cause passengers to be thrown about in the passenger compartments, opening the possibility of injury. Emergency braking procedures are generally considered to be a last resort. For these reasons, penalty applications of the emergency brake triggered by the alerter, ATP, or programmed stop systems should be avoided whenever possible.

System Operation — Communications

Communications in the high-speed rail simulation system is via a broadcast text-based system. An operator in each vehicle, as well as the CTC operator, can enter messages through the computer keyboard. When the message is completed (either with a carriage return or when the message length reaches 80 characters), it is sent out over the network and received by all other active simulation elements. Thus, everybody hears everybody.

The protocol used for these communications aids in reducing any confusion in the messages. Specifically, the message sender identifies the intended recipient of the message, adds the body of the message, and terminates with self-identification. All identification is with vehicle identifiers (vehicle ID numbers are issued when the operator starts a shift).

For example, the following exchange might take place between the CTC and a train operator in vehicle E48401:

"E48401, request position, CTC."

"CTC, block 5, kmpost 11, destination East Station, E48401."

In this exchange, the CTC operator requests a position update from operator E48401, who responded with a summary of the current vehicle position. All of the active vehicles in the simulation heard this exchange. The exchange format could be shortened to the following, without any loss of information:

"E48401, req pos, CTC."

"CTC, blk 5, km 11, dest E St, E48401."

Tables A-4 and A-5 contain a summary of the most frequently used messages and responses used in the system. Although any text is allowable, these tables summarize the set of the most frequently used messages and responses, in shorthand form to minimize the necessary typing.

Most of the messages included in these tables represent typical information, which might be conveyed between a vehicle operator and a CTC operator in an operational rail system. In a typical rail system, there is very limited provision for exchange of data between vehicles and centralized control. Although this is changing as technology progresses, voice communications over radio still represent a significant method for transferring state information between the vehicles and the CTC.[3]

System Operation — Schedules

During a shift of operation, the vehicle operator is required to make three round trips in the shuttle operation. Each round trip starts at West Station, proceeds to East Station, reverses direction, and returns to West Station. Each trip leg (one-way) is scheduled to take twenty minutes. When the train reaches the destination station, the vehicle is stopped and the doors are opened for a period of one minute, to allow the passengers onboard to disembark. The train is then routed around the reversing loop to change direction. The looping procedure requires approximately seven minutes. When the train arrives at the same station in the opposite direction, it is again stopped, and the doors are again opened for a period of two minutes, to allow new passengers to board. The total scheduled round trip time is one hour. A printed schedule is provided to the operator for each shift.

---

[3] A complex keyboard was used for communications instead of the radio so that the communications could be easily recorded for analysis following an experiment.

Table A-4. Standard Communications Message Initiated by Vehicle Operator

Messages Initiated by Vehicle Operator	Message Shorthand Form	Response From CTC Operator
announce departure	"CTC, depart \<station>, \<vehID>"	"\<vehID>, ack depart \<station>, CTC"
announce arrival	"CTC, arrive \<station>, \<vehID>"	"\<vehID>, ack arrive \<station>, CTC"
inform of vehicle failure	"CTC, \<brake | motor> fail, fixed, \<vehID>"	"\<vehID>, ack fail, CTC"
inform of obstruction	"CTC, obstruct at \<cross num>, \<vehID>"	"\<vehID>, ack obstruct, CTC"
inform of collision	"CTC, collide at \<cross num>, \<vehID>"	"\<vehID>, ack collide, CTC"
request break	"CTC, req break at \<station>, \<vehID>"	"\<vehID>, break req accept, CTC" "\<vehID>, break req deny, CTC"

Table A-5. Standard Communications Messages Initiated by CTC Operator

Messages Initiated by CTC Operator	Message Shorthand Form	Response From Vehicle Operator
request vehicle position	"\<vehID>, req pos, CTC"	"CTC, km \<num>, \<vehID>"
request vehicle status	"\<vehID>, req veh status, CTC"	"CTC, status OK, \<vehID>" "CTC, \<brake|motor> fail, \<vehID>" "CTC, obstruct at \<cross>, \<vehID>" "CTC, collide at \<cross>, \<vehID>"
request automation mode status	"\<vehID>, req mode status, CTC"	"CTC, man mode, \<vehID>" "CTC, cruise mode, \<vehID>" "CTC, pstop mode, \<vehID>" "CTC, auto mode, \<vehID>"

Under certain circumstances, there may be deviations from the prescribed schedule. In this case, it is the responsibility of the CTC operator to adjust the schedules accordingly. The vehicle operator must wait for CTC instructions before departing a station at any time that is not in compliance with the prescribed schedule.

System Operation — Role of CTC Operator

The central traffic control operator (CTC operator) is the coordinating element in the rail system. The operator must monitor the positions and speeds (when possible) of the vehicles in the system, and adjust operating parameters of the system in order to achieve the system goals. The CTC operator also represents the coordination point between the vehicles, as well as with "outside" agencies (such as fire, police, power, maintenance, etc.).

Given this perspective, the CTC operators have a level of jurisdiction that is higher than the wayside signals, the operating rules, and any other influence. In short, when there is a conflict between influences that govern the action taken by a vehicle operator, the CTC operator is always the highest authority. Therefore, CTC operators are supervisors, with respect to the vehicle operators, and vehicle operators are required to follow all directions given by the CTC operators. This supervisory role has a higher level of responsibility than the task of monitoring.

System Operation — Obstruction Hazards

As mentioned in the braking performance section, the track used in the simulation system has **highway grade crossings**. These are points in the rail system where highway roads and rail tracks intersect. In total, there are five grade crossings, one each located in blocks 0, 1, 11, 12, and 13. At each grade crossing, highway vehicles (cars) can cross in front of the train from either direction. These vehicles are visible at over a half-kilometer distance.

In each of the blocks containing grade crossings, there is a civil speed limit of 62.1 mph (100 km/h). This means that, regardless of the signal level in the block, the maximum speed of a vehicle in the block is 62.1 mph (100 km/h). The ATP system is programmed to detect when these blocks are entered, and will use this civil speed limit in its restriction rules.

Traffic at the grade crossings arrives according to a probabilistic process.[4] A car will proceed across the crossing only if there is sufficient distance to clear the crossing before the train. (In other words, a car will not proceed if there is not enough room.) However, it is possible for a car to become disabled as it is crossing the tracks, which will result in an obstruction for the train. In this event, the train operator must bring the train to a stop before the intersection. If the train is not stopped in time, a collision will occur, which will be indicated by a cracked windscreen.

It is important that the train operator be able to quickly assess the crossing traffic and determine whether the train must be stopped. On one hand, a collision is a major event, and will result in a significant delay in operation. On the other hand, stopping the train unnecessarily will also cause delays in service. It is up to the vehicle operator to evaluate the situation and determine the best course of action under these constraints.

If a collision occurs, the vehicle operator must stop the vehicle and immediately contact the CTC operator to report the collision. In the case of a collision, the windscreen will appear "cracked."

---

[4] There wasn't a good way to model the motorist's motivation and the frequency with which the motorist crosses in front of the train. We addressed this problem by making a simplifying assumption and modeling the outcome of the motorist's behavior based upon a probabilistic process. This probabilistic process was intended to cover all the cases in which the motorist may or may not cross in front of the train.

This crack will remain for the remainder of the shift. For each of three collisions that might occur within a shift, the windscreen will become progressively more "cracked."

System Operation — Operator Performance Requirements

In order to assure that each vehicle operator is capable of adequately controlling the train, the performance of each operator (test subject) is monitored throughout the test sessions. As an incentive, there is a bonus system that provides monetary rewards for good performance. If operator performance does not fall within certain minimum criteria, penalties may be assessed. At the end of each experiment session, the subject's performance is evaluated with regard to bonuses and penalties.

By decree of the Federal Code of Regulations, Number 49, Part 240, the performance of rail vehicle operators (locomotive engineers) is regulated such that any willful violation of speed restrictions or signal indications is punishable with both a monetary fine and a loss of certification (which may be permanent or temporary, depending on the circumstances). The monetary fines are substantial, and can range from a minimum of $250 to a maximum of $20,000. In short, these violations are considered serious offenses, and are not tolerated.

Because of these regulations, speed and signal compliance are considered key performance items. In the simulation system, violations are defined by ATP-induced or signal-induced penalty applications of the emergency brakes. During the road test period of the training phase, such a violation will result in disqualification of the subject from further participation. In this case, the subject will be paid for training period. During the experiment phase, the first violation in a shift will result in a penalty of 100,000 bonus points. If a second violation occurs in the same shift, the subject will be disqualified from further participation in the experiment. In this case, payment will cover the sessions that have been completed to date.

In addition, willful circumvention of the vehicle safety systems, such as the alerter system, will not be tolerated. If a subject is found to have bypassed these safety systems, the subject will not be permitted to complete the experimental tests. In this case, payment will cover the sessions that have been completed to date.

Other key operator performance items include station stopping accuracy, schedule maintenance, and response to emergency (or failure) situations. In general, good performance in these areas will result in the award of bonus points, which result in an increase in payment for that session. The bonus point's schedules are shown in Tables A-6 and A-7, and the penalty point's schedules are shown in Tables A-8 through A-10.

Table A-6 shows the bonus points that result from station stopping performance. The stopping point is defined as the first point at which the vehicle stops, in the vicinity of the station. The closer the stop occurs to the designated stopping point, the more bonus points are awarded. The bonus points are distributed to favor undershoot (i.e., it's preferable to stop before the designated point than after). Figure A-7 shows this relationship in graphical form.

Table A-6. Bonus Point Schedule for Station Stopping Accuracy

station stop accuracy	bonus points
more than 10m before stop point deviation < -10.0 (undershoot)	0
-10.0 <= deviation < -8.0	+400
-8.0 <= deviation < -6.0	+800
-6.0 <= deviation < -4.0	+1200
-4.0 <= deviation < -2.0	+1600
-2.0 <= dev <= +2.0	+2000
+2.0 < deviation <= +3.0	+1600
+3.0 < deviation <= +4.0	+1200
+4.0 < deviation <= +5.0	+800
+5.0 < deviation <= +6.0	+400
more than 6m beyond stop point +6.0 < deviation (overshoot)	0

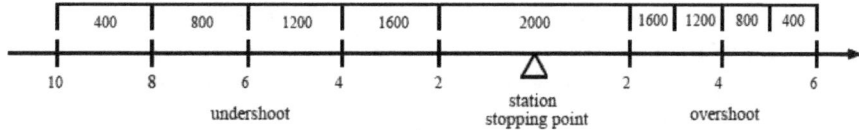

Figure A-7. Bonus Point Diagram for Station Stopping Accuracy

Table A-7 shows the bonus points that result from schedule accuracy. Because there may be emergency situations that will affect schedule maintenance (such as an obstruction or collision), the schedule is adjusted for such occurrences. As with station stopping accuracy, the bonus point distribution shows a preference for early arrivals over late arrivals. Although the bias fosters early arrivals over late arrivals, this bias is small relative to the total number of points the participant could earn. This bias is countered by penalties for going too fast through overspeed protection. If the engineer speeds, a penalty brake application is applied which results in a schedule delay far in excess of the benefits of speeding. A graphical representation is shown in Figure A-8.

Table A-8 shows the bonus point schedule associated with failure and emergency response. In general, you are evaluated in terms of the response time to the failure, as well as the accuracy ("correctness") of the first response action. The actual events used to evaluate the accuracy depend on the specific emergency being evaluated. A summary of these appears in the bottom portion of Table A-8.

Table A-7. Bonus Point Schedule for Schedule Accuracy

schedule accuracy	bonus points
more than 26 secs early deviation < -26.0	0
-26.0 <= deviation < -22.0	+400
-22.0 <= deviation < -18.0	+800
-18.0 <= deviation < -14.0	+1200
-14.0 <= deviation < -10.0	+1600
-10.0 <= deviation <= +8.0	+2000
+8.0 < deviation <= +12.0	+1600
+12.0 < deviation <= +16.0	+1200
+16.0 < deviation <= +20.0	+800
+20.0 < deviation <= +24.0	+400
more than 24 secs late +24.0 < deviation	0

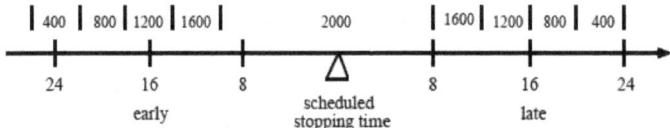

Figure A-8. Bonus Point Diagram for Schedule Accuracy

Table A-8. Bonus/Penalty Point Schedule for Emergency Response

Emergency response time (sec)	bonus points
less than 2.0	+1000
more than 2.0, less than 5.0	+750
more than 5.0, less than 10.0	+500
more than 10.0, less than 20.0	+250
more than 20.0	0
first response accuracy, obstruction	**bonus/penalty points**
correct braking action	+1000
incorrect braking action	+500
error (other command action)	0
safety hazard (door open command)	-1000

first response accuracy, brake failure	bonus/penalty points
correct action (switch brake pump)	+1000
incorrect command action	0
safety hazard (estop, door open commands)	-1000

first response accuracy, motor failure	bonus/penalty points
correct action (brake, then reset failed motor)	+1000
partially correct action (depress reset button for wrong motor, failure to apply brakes first)	+500
incorrect command action	0
safety hazard (estop, door open commands)	-1000

Tables A-9 and A-10 show the penalties that can be levied for poor performance. Table A-9 identifies penalties that result from explicit violations of the operating rules. The most significant is a penalty application of the emergency brakes, resulting from either a speed violation (via the ATP system) or a signal violation. Both of these are considered serious offenses, and the resultant penalty is substantial. The next penalty is for opening the passenger doors when the vehicle is outside the station. This action is considered a serious compromise of passenger safety, and is penalized accordingly. The third penalty is for unnecessary use of the emergency brake. Use of the emergency brake takes a heavy mechanical toll on the train systems, and results in a very uncomfortable ride for the passengers. Gratuitous use of the emergency brake is inappropriate, and the penalty for unnecessary use is significant enough to outweigh any benefit that might be obtained (such as improving the station stopping or schedule accuracy). The fourth penalty is imposed if the operator fails to stop the vehicle within the station. In this event, the doors must not be opened. In addition, the vehicle operator must notify the CTC operator of the situation, and await further instructions from the CTC operator.

Table A-9. Penalty Point Schedule for Violations

infraction	penalty points
Penalty application for speed compliance (ATP) or signal compliance violation	-50,000
Passenger doors opened outside of station bounds (more than 20m undershoot or 100m overshoot)	-10,000
Unnecessary application of emergency brake (no emergency present)	-5,000
Station overrun	-2,000

Table A-10 shows the penalty points that occur if there is a collision with a highway vehicle at a grade crossing. The intent of this schedule is to impart a sense that collisions at higher velocities are more serious—in the event that a collision is inevitable, the operator should do as much as possible to reduce the impact of that collision by reducing the vehicle as much as possible.

Table A-10. Penalty Point Schedule for Grade Crossing Collisions

collision impact speed (mph)	penalty points
Between 37.3 and 62.1 mph (60 and 100 km/h)	-1000
Between 24.9 and 37.3 mph (40 and 60 km/h)	-750
Between 12.4 and 24.9 mph (20 and 40 km/h)	-500
Between 0 and 12.4 mph (20 km/h)	-250

After the total bonus points are computed for a shift, the bonus points are converted into a pay bonus, at the rate of one dollar for each ten thousand points. There are a total of eleven station stops per shift, for a maximum possible 44,000 points per shift for station stopping performance. Because the number of failures and obstructions will vary from shift to shift, it is not possible to determine beforehand the maximum possible bonus points that are available. However, in most cases, there will be sufficient opportunity for an excess of 50,000 bonus points, which will yield an equivalent pay rate in excess of $10 per hour.

APPENDIX B. WRITTEN REVIEW QUIZ

Instructions: For each question, circle the letter of the answer you feel best answers the question.

1. "Kilometer posts" are located where?

    a) on the wayside, at tenth-kilometer intervals

    b) on the vehicle instrument panel

    c) on the wayside, at kilometer intervals

    d) on a monitor screen in the CTC operations center

2. Which of the following is considered an automatic mode?

    a) programmed stop

    b) emergency stop

    c) ATP warning

    d) alerter warning

3. If the signal level of the upcoming block is full yellow (YYY), what is the speed limit in that block?

    a) 15 km/h (9.3 mph)

    b) 150 km/h (93.2 mph)

    c) 80 km/h (49.7 mph)

    d) 230 km/h (142.9 mph)

4. What is the expected one-way travel time between East Station and West Station?

    a) 5 minutes

    b) 20 minutes

    c) 15 minutes

    d) 25 minutes

5. How many signal levels are used?

    a) one

    b) seven

    c) four

    d) five

6. How many control modes are available on the train?

    a) none

    b) four

    c) three

    d) ten

7. When full service braking is applied, what is the typical tank pressure?

    a) 1000 psi

    b) 100 psi

    c) 0 psi

    d) 22 psi

8. Where are block signals located?

    a) at the entrance to every block

    b) in the middle of every block

    c) every 50 m (164 ft)

    d) on the back of the preceding train

9. What is the expected distance to accelerate to 300 km/h from a standing stop on level ground?

    a) 11.5 km (7.1 mi)

    b) 21.2 km (13.2 mi)

    c) 4.5 km (2.8 mi)

    d) 5.7 km (3.5 mi)

10. Which category best describes the type of system being operated?

    a) shuttle service

    b) subway

    c) commuter rail

    d) long-haul freight

11. There are four electric traction motors. How many circuit breakers in total are used to protect these traction motors?

    a) eight

    b) four

    c) one

    d) none

12. How is the programmed stop mode disabled?

    a) by manually applying the brakes

    b) by depressing the cruise control enable button

    c) by depressing the programmed stop enable button

    d) by waiting until the vehicle comes to a stop

13. During system operation, how many trains are simultaneously in use?

    a) four

    b) one

    c) ten

    d) two

14. In autopilot mode, the control system maintains the proper speed through which control mechanism?

    a) thrust only

    b) braking only

    c) both thrust and braking

    d) magnetic levitation

15. How is the cruise control mode enabled?

    a) by depressing the cruise control button while braking to the desired speed

    b) by depressing autopilot and cruise control buttons simultaneously

    c) by holding the vehicle at a steady speed under manual control

    d) by depressing the cruise control button while traveling at the desired speed

16. What is the relative status of the CTC operator, from the perspective of a train operator?

    a) supervisor

    b) subordinate

    c) monitor

    d) peer

17. If the vehicle speed exceeds the maximum allowable speed by more than 15 km/h, the ATP system does what?

   a) applies the emergency brake

   b) applies more thrust

   c) limits the effectiveness of manual thrust commands

   d) applies the service brake

18. What is the purpose of the block signal system?

   a) for vehicle operator to determine the number of vehicles allowed in the block

   b) for vehicle operator to determine the maximum allowable speed in the block

   c) give vehicle operators something to do

   d) for vehicle operator to determine the number of passengers allowed on board

19. In a block signaling system, how many trains are allowed to occupy a single block at the same time?

   a) two

   b) four

   c) none

   d) one

20. How many different braking modes are available to the vehicle operator?

   a) one

   b) three

   c) five

   d) two

21. If the vehicle operator moves the vehicle when the doors are still open, what happens?

    a) the motor circuit breakers are tripped

    b) the passengers are warned over the intercom

    c) the emergency brakes are applied

    d) the doors close automatically

22. What is the expected stopping distance from 300 km/h (186.4 mph) to 100 km/h (62.1 mph) under full-service braking on level ground?

    a) 21.2 km (13.2 mi)

    b) 11.5 km (7.1 mi)

    c) 4.5 km (2.8 mi)

    d) 5.7 km (3.5 mi)

23. What warning does the alerter system give the vehicle operator before a penalty application is imposed?

    a) chime only, for 5 seconds

    b) electric shock through the seat, for 5 seconds

    c) flashing light only, for 15 seconds

    d) flashing lights and chime, for 10 seconds

24. How does the vehicle operator know the speed of the train?

    a) from the CTC operator

    b) from the speedometer, on the vehicle instrument panel

    c) from the brake pressure gauge, on the vehicle instrument panel

    d) from the block signaling system

25. Where are CTC operators located?

   a) in a maintenance shed

   b) in small booths along the wayside

   c) in a centralized operations center

   d) in the last car of each train

APPENDIX C. TRAIN SCHEDULE

00:05:00	Depart West Station
00:23:30	Arrive East Station — discharge passengers
00:26:00	Depart East Station — loop around
00:33:00	Arrive East Station — board passengers
00:35:00	Depart East Station
00:53:00	Arrive West Station — discharge passengers
00:56:00	Depart West Station — loop around
01:03:00	Arrive West Station — board passengers
01:05:00	Depart West Station
01:23:30	Arrive East Station — discharge passengers
01:26:00	Depart East Station — loop around
01:33:00	Arrive East Station — board passengers
01:35:00	Depart East Station
01:53:00	Arrive West Station — discharge passengers
01:56:00	Depart West Station — loop around
02:03:00	Arrive West Station — board passengers
02:05:00	Depart West Station
02:23:30	Arrive East Station — discharge passengers
02:26:00	Depart East Station — loop around
02:33:00	Arrive East Station — board passengers
02:35:00	Depart East Station
02:53:00	Arrive West Station — discharge passengers

APPENDIX D. EXIT QUESTIONNAIRE

Please answer the following questions.

1. Rate the levels of automation in order of preference (use "1" for the automation level you liked the most, "3" for the automation level you liked the least)?

   __ full automation (autopilot)

   __ partial automation (cruise control and programmed stop)

   __ no automation (manual control)

2. Rate the levels of automation according to level of "awareness" (use "1" for the automation level in which you felt the most aware, "3" for the automation level in which you felt the least aware)?

   __ full automation (autopilot)

   __ partial automation (cruise control and programmed stop)

   __ no automation (manual control)

3. Do you feel that the training process provided adequate preparation for the test task?

   __ yes __ no

4. Any other comments? Critical comments are appreciated.

APPENDIX E. INTERACTIVE TRAINING PROCEDURE

The subject training takes place over two 3-hour sessions. Prior to the first session, the subjects are instructed to review the training tutorial material, in preparation for a written quiz. The first training session should begin with the subject completing this written review quiz. This quiz consists of 25 multiple choice questions, and is intended to be on the level of a written quiz given by a state driver licensing department. The quiz is used to provide motivation for the subjects to review the tutorial material, and to allow the instructor to identify any weakness areas prior to the interactive training.

The first session continues with the interactive segment. The instructor briefly introduces the subject to the CTC display, and explains the role of the CTC operator with respect to overall system operation. The instructor then introduces the subject to the train simulator, and reviews the basics of operation in the following order:

1. Identify the OTW viewport and all visual cues that appear in this display

2. Identify the instrument panel display and all of the instruments that appear on that display

3. Identify the combined control lever

4. Identify the keyboard controls

5. Have the subject move the train slowly out of the station, noting behavior of the head-up display

6. Test operation of the alerter system

7. Test operation of the ATP system

8. Make note of grade crossing details, mile posts, block signals, landmarks

9. Describe operation of cruise control, test

10. Describe operation of autopilot, test

11. Describe operation of programmed stop, test, and

12. Describe procedure for stopping in station, coach through the procedure.

The first training session continues with two round trips. In effect, this is the first opportunity for the subject to experience solo operation, with the instructor acting as CTC controller. On the first, the goal is to familiarize the subject with use of the automation modes, as well as the operating schedule and interaction with the CTC operator. The subject is instructed to use manual control for the first trip leg, cruise control and programmed stop in the loop, and autopilot on the return trip leg. On the second round trip, the goal is to familiarize the subject with the failure modes. The subject is instructed to use manual control for the entire trip, and experiences a series of expected failures that require operator response.

The second training session represents a combination practice session and road test. The subjects are instructed to treat this session as a real shift of operation. They are to operate the train in manual mode, and are to adhere to the schedule to the best of their abilities. The first round trip (i.e., the first four station stops) is a practice period, and the remaining time is a road test. Their proficiency is judged on the basis of their station stopping accuracy.

REFERENCES

Askey, Shumei Y. (1995). Design and Evaluation of Decision Aids for Control of High-Speed Trains: Experiments and Model. Ph.D. Thesis, Massachusetts Institute of Technology, Cambridge, MA.

Askey, Shumei Y., and. Sheridan, Thomas (1996). *Safety of High-Speed Guided Ground Transportation Systems, Phase II: Design and Evaluation of Decision Aids for Control of High-Speed Trains: Experiments and Model*. Report No. DOT/FRA/ORD-96/09. Washington, DC: U.S. Department of Transportation, Federal Railroad Administration.

Bing, Alan J. (1990). *An Assessment of High-Speed Rail Safety Issues and Research Needs*. Washington, DC: U.S. Department of Transportation, Federal Railroad Administration.

Endsley, M. (1987). SAGAT: A methodology for the measurement of situation awareness (NOR DOC 87-83). Hawthorne, CA: Northrup Corp.

Endsley, M. (1988). Situation Awareness Global Assessment Technique (SAGAT). In Proceedings of the National Aerospace and Electronics Conference. New York: IEEE.

Endsley, M. (1995). Toward a Theory of Situation Awareness in Dynamic Systems. *Human Factors*, Vol. 37 (1), 32-64.

Gaba, David M., Howard, Steven K., and Small, Stephen D. (1995). Situation Awareness in Anesthesiology. *Human Factors*, Vol. 37(1), 20-31.

Goldstein, I., and Dorfman P. (1978). Speed stress and load stress as determinants of performance in a time-sharing task. *Human Factors*, Vol. 20.

Hald, A. (1952). *Statistical Theory with Engineering Applications*. New York: John Wiley & Sons.

Hamburg, Morris, and Young, Peg (1994). *Statistical Analysis for Decision Making* (Sixth Edition). Orlando, Florida: Dryden Press.

Hendy, K.C. (1995) Situation Awareness and Workload: Birds of a Feather? Advisory Group for Aerospace Research and Development (AGARD) Conference Proceedings 575. Presented at American Medical Panel Symposium on "Situational Awareness: Limitations and Enhancements in the Aviation Environment," Brussels, Belgium, April 1995.

Lanzilotta, Edward J. (1996). "Dynamic Risk Estimation: Development of the Safety State Model and Experimental Application to High-Speed Rail Operation," Ph.D. Thesis, Massachusetts Institute of Technology, Cambridge, MA.

Moray, N. (1986). Monitoring Behavior and Supervisory Control. In Boff, Kaufman, Thomas, *Handbook of Perception and Human Performance*, Volume II. New York: John Wiley and Sons.

Parasuraman, R. (1986). Vigilance, Monitoring, and Search. In Boff, Kaufman, Thomas, *Handbook of Perception and Human Performance*, Volume II. New York: John Wiley and Sons.

Sanders, Mark S., and McCormick, Ernest J. (1987). *Human Factors in Engineering and Design* (Second Edition). New York: McGraw-Hill.

Sarter, Nadine B., and Woods, David D. (1995). How in the World Did We Ever Get into That Mode? Mode Error and Awareness in Supervisory Control. Human Factors (37)1, pp. 5-19.

Senders, J. (1964). The Human Operator as a Monitor and Controller of Multidegree of Freedom Systems. IEEE Trans. on Human Factors in Electronics, Vol. HFE-5, No. 1.

Sheridan, Thomas B., Lanzilotta, Edward J., and Askey, Shumei Y. (1994). *Safety of High-Speed Guided Ground Transportation Systems, Phase I: Function Analysis and Theoretical Considerations*. Report No. DOT/FRA/ORD-94/24. Washington, DC: US Department of Transportation, Federal Railroad Administration.

Smith, Kip., and Hancock, P.A. (1995). Situation Awareness is Adaptive, Externally Directed Consciousness. *Human Factors* Vol. 37 (1), pp. 137-148.

Tukey, John W. (1977). *Exploratory Data Analysis*. Reading, MA: Addison-Wesley.

Wickens, C. (1992). *Engineering Psychology and Human Performance* (Second Edition). New York: Harper-Collins.